THE ESSENTIAL BOOK OF TR MEDICINE
VOLUME

THE ESSENTIAL BOOK
OF
TRADITIONAL CHINESE
MEDICINE

VOLUME I: THEORY

LIU YANCHI

Translated by
FANG TINGYU *and* CHEN LAIDI

Written and Edited in Collaboration with
KATHLEEN VIAN *and* PETER ECKMAN

New York
COLUMBIA UNIVERSITY PRESS
1988

The illustrations on the jacket and within the text were specially commissioned for this volume and drawn by Cheng Duoduo.

Library of Congress Cataloging-in-Publication Data

Liu, Yen-ch'ih (Liu Yanchi)
The essential book of traditional Chinese medicine.

Includes bibliographies and index.
Contents: v. 1. Theory.
1. Medicine, Chinese.   I. Vian, Kathleen.
II. Eckman, Peter.   III. Title.   [DNLM: 1. Medicine,
Oriental Traditional—China. WB 50 JC6 L85e]
R601.L713   1987   610   87-10349
ISBN 0-231-06520-5 (set)
ISBN 0-231-06196-X (v. 1)
ISBN 0-231-06518-3 (v. 2)
ISBN 0-231-10357-3 (v. 1, pbk.)
ISBN 0-231-10359-X (v. 2, pbk.)

Columbia University Press
New York   Chichester, West Sussex
Copyright © 1988, 1995 Columbia University Press and
The People's Medical Publishing House

Printed in the United States of America

p 10 9 8 7 6 5 4 3 2

This book is a joint effort of
The People's Medical Publishing House
(Beijing)
and
The United States–China Educational Institute
(San Francisco)

Supported by
The Educational Foundation of America
(Westport, Connecticut)

CONTENTS

FOREWORD

　　中國傳統醫學是中國人民長期與疾病做鬥爭的智慧結晶，內容豐富，源遠流長。它具有獨特的理論體系和豐富的臨床實踐經驗，千百年來爲中華民族的繁衍昌盛做出了貢獻。西方醫藥界不少人士對中國傳統醫學具有濃厚興趣，美中教育學院、人民衛生出版社、哥倫比亞大學出版社組織了有關專家，合作出版了這本《中醫入門》。這本書肯定會增進西方對中國傳統醫學的瞭解。我祝願通過這樣的橋樑，中美醫學交流將取得巨大成功。

崔月犁
中國衛生部部長

FOREWORD

Traditional Chinese medicine is the crystal of wisdom of the Chinese people in their long period of struggle against diseases. Its content is substantial and it is of long standing and well established. It has its own theoretical system and rich clinical experience, having made contributions to the prosperous growth of the Chinese nation in the past thousands of years. Many of the figures in the Western medical world have found traditional Chinese medicine interesting. The United States–China Educational Institute, the Peoples' Medical Publishing House, and Columbia University Press have solicited a group of experts to publish cooperatively this *Essential Book of Traditional Chinese Medicine.* It is expected that this book will enhance the understanding of traditional Chinese medicine in the Western world. It is hoped that the exchange in medical science between the United States and China will result in great successes through such a bridge.

Cui Yueli
Minister of Public Health,
People's Republic of China

ACKNOWLEDGMENTS

The writing and production of *The Essential Book of Traditional Chinese Medicine* began over six years ago with a decision between the People's Medical Publishing House and the United States–China Educational Institute to cooperate together on this project. But the credit for these two volumes really should be given to all the traditional Chinese medical scholars who have contributed to this extraordinary body of knowledge for over 4,000 years. The Ministry of Public Health of the People's Republic of China should also be acknowledged for their foresight in organizing a system of institutions for the understanding and the development of traditional Chinese medicine.

For over four thousand years, scholars and medical practitioners have documented the ways of maintaining health and treating illness through the use of herbs, acupuncture, and intelligent life-style practices. As early as 4000 B.C, there were legends about Shen Nong, who tasted hundreds of herbs before they were used medicinally. During the third century B.C., the *Classic of Internal Medicine,* an eighteen-volume document, laid the theoretical foundation for traditional Chinese medicine and it is considered to be one of the greatest medical classics in China. Hua Tuo, a renowned surgeon in the third century A.D., was the first practitioner in China to perform operations under local anesthesia. Yang Jizhou, a prominent acupuncturist during the Ming dynasty, compiled the *Compendium of Acupuncture and Moxibustion,* a work that is still revered by modern acupuncturists.

The human body is a fascinating and intricate system and Chinese scholars have long been studying the ways of conceptualizing the body, with its abundance of energy and physiological activities, and of promoting its health. The gathering of information about the functions of the human body and how to treat illnesses for many thousands of years is an impressive accomplishment and it has resulted in traditional Chinese medicine permeating into the consciousness of the Chinese people. It has become a cornerstone in the foundation of Chinese culture. Today, people think about their health as a balance of the person and the environment, the active and the receptive.

In 1954, the Chinese Ministry of Public Health decided to undertake a major effort to systematically organize this body of knowledge, and it has resulted in some impressive achievements. Its policy was to combine the resources and experiences of traditional Chinese doctors with those of Chinese scientists and physicians who are trained in Western medicine, and to channel this intellectual energy into developing traditional Chinese medicine. The Chinese Ministry of Public Health broadened its base of information by organizing scholars to research historical documents. Two-year postgraduate training programs in traditional Chinese medicine were designed for Chinese physicians trained in Western medicine. Research scientists were encouraged to investigate specific research agendas related to traditional Chinese medicine and its integration with Western medicine. Finally, the Ministry of Public Health developed a policy to protect and improve the resources of Chinese medicinal herbs.

To implement these policies, the Ministry established a Bureau of Traditional Medicine within its organization and departments of traditional Chinese medicine in every province and autonomous region in China. In the late 1950s, the Academy of Traditional Chinese Medicine was set up in Beijing, and colleges of traditional Chinese medicine and research institutes were organized in most provinces and autonomous regions. Currently, China has 300,000 doctors and paraprofessionals of traditional Chinese medicine. There are more than 1,100 hospitals of traditional Chinese medicine and some 9,000 general hospitals nationwide which have departments of traditional Chinese medicine. Most recently, the Ministry of Public Health announced plans to step up the training of doctors of traditional medicine so that by 1990 there will be three such doctors for every ten thousand people as compared to only one per ten thousand at the moment.

This enormous undertaking by the Ministry of Public Health to develop traditional Chinese medicine is leading to improved health care practices, new scientific breakthroughs, and a greater understanding and interest in this field among people all over the world. To provide Western health practitioners and scientists with updated information about traditional Chinese medicine and to stimulate the integration of traditional Chinese medicine with Western medicine, the People's Medical Publishing House of the Ministry of Public Health and the United States–China Educational Institute decided to cooperate on the production of *The Essential Book of Traditional Chinese Medicine,* volumes 1 and 2.

This project was made possible by a grant from the Educational Foundation of America, and we are deeply appreciative of its support. Producing *The Essential Book of Traditional Chinese Medicine,* volumes 1 and 2, was a major undertaking that could not have been realized without the full support and confidence given to us by Richard and Sharon Ettinger, Cyrus and Elaine Hapood, Barbara Ettinger, Robert Kalinonski, Edward Anderson, Richard Hansen, and the other members of the Board of Trustees of the Educational Foundation of America.

The People's Medical Publishing House was responsible for determining the author to write about the theory and the clinical practice of traditional Chinese medicine. It was also responsible for identifying the experts to do the translation work. The United States–China Educational Institute would edit and, in some cases, would add to, the manuscript in a way that would preserve the intentions of the author while making changes that would help Westerners understand what the author intended. The editing would also preserve the integrity of the Chinese culture represented in the writing and develop a style that is familiar to the Western mind. These were the principles used by the staff of the Institute.

We thought that if information about the theoretical and the practical components of traditional Chinese medicine were presented in a manner that was readily understood in the West, it might enhance the practice of traditional Chinese medicine in the West and foster more interest in the West in cooperative research activities with Chinese scientists. There would also be an opportunity to synthesize the knowledge and experiences of both Chinese and Western medicine, and we were very much interested in encouraging this kind of synthesis.

Over the last five years, the Chinese portion of this project has been administered by Vice-President Wang Shuqi of the People's

Medical Publishing House. After he transferred to the Peking Union Medical College, the project was led by Vice-President Dong Mianguo. Their dedication and untiring energy in solving problems which arose during our cooperation have impressed the staff of the United States—China Educational Institute. Dr. Liu Yanchi has a distinguished career as associate professor at the Beijing College of Traditional Chinese Medicine. He is currently head of the Teaching Section of Basic Theory of Traditional Chinese Medicine and is on the editing commissions of the *Chinese Medical Encyclopedia* and the *Digest of Traditional Chinese Medicine*. Mr. Fang Tingyu and Ms. Chen Laidi, chosen as the translators, have much experience in translation work. Mr. Xu Wei and Ms. Chang Zexun, editors at the People's Medical Publishing House, provided valuable assistance and carried out their responsibilities remarkably well. Dr. Ou Mujie and Ms. Nissi Wang reviewed the manuscripts and meticulously and conscientiously ensured that the thinking and the clinical practices were written, translated, and edited with accuracy and integrity. Nissi Wang, a Chinese-American at the People's Medical Publishing House in Beijing, has played an invaluable role in the development of these two volumes. In fact, all these scholars at the People's Medical Publishing House and the Beijing College of Traditional Chinese Medicine played a vital role in transmitting the knowledge and experiences of traditional Chinese medicine to the West.

The main task of the Institute was to communicate effectively in English the concepts and the treatment modalities of traditional Chinese medicine. This was an extremely complicated process and required agile and creative minds with sensitivity to both cultures. Our editors and collaborators needed to understand the Chinese way of thinking and to communicate these concepts in a format that was easily understood in the West. We were fortunate to have Kathleen Vian, Ph.D., and Dr. Peter Eckman, who collaborated with Dr. Liu Yanchi in the writing and editing of the first volume, on the theoretical aspects of traditional Chinese medicine. Dr. Vian applied her unique sensitivity to and understanding of traditional Chinese medicine and Chinese culture, and she effectively communicated these concepts in the English language. Dr. Peter Eckman, a graduate of New York University, where he received both an M.D. and a Ph.D. in physiology, has devoted over ten years to the study, practice, and teaching of traditional Chinese medicine, which is now the focus of his professional life. The editorial consultant for Dr. Liu's volume on clinical practice was Barbara Gastel, M.D., M.P.H. Dr. Gastel has distinguished herself as a scientific writer who spent two years in Beijing as a Fellow of the United States–China Educational Institute teaching scientific writing and communication to medical scholars at Beijing Medical University and at the *Chinese Medical Journal.* Prior to her work in Beijing, she was an assistant professor in the Writing Program of the Massachusetts Institute of Technology. While Dr. Gastel was in Beijing, she worked with Nissi Wang and the staff of the People's Medical Publishing House in editing volume 2 of *The Essential Book of Traditional Chinese Medicine.* Drs. Vian and Gastel are some of the most intellectually talented writers that we have had the privilege to know, and they have an abundance of respect for traditional Chinese medicine and culture. They spent many hours writing and rewriting this manuscript. To them, we express our indebtedness and our appreciation.

Early in our discussions with the administrators of the People's Medical Publishing House, we realized the importance of communicating the concepts of traditional Chinese medicine through visual means. The Institute sought the assistance of Mr. Cheng Duoduo, who is a talented painter from Shanghai. We also sought out the assistance of Mrs. Sally Yu Leung, a sensitive and thoughtful Chinese-American, who provided unending assistance in the development of the illustrations. Mr. Cheng and Mrs. Yu Leung were attracted to the issue of how to communicate traditional Chinese concepts to Westerners and they accepted this assignment with a great deal of interest. All the illustrations were painted with a Chinese brush technique called *bai miao* or Chinese brush-line drawing. As you will see, the beginning of each chapter has Mr. Cheng's illustrations which summarize the concept of each chapter. He paints with unusual sensitivity and imagination, two qualities which are so essential to promoting communication and understanding about traditional Chinese medicine.

Many of us who have worked on this project were inspired to initiate the production of *The Essential Book of Traditional Chinese Medicine* by our association with Jennifer Mei, Dr. Sadja Greenwood, and Dr. Ho Wingtong at the Min An Health Center. Min An is a community health facility located in San Francisco's Chinatown. At Min An, Western and traditional Chinese practitioners work side by side. Together they provide a variety of health services, including women's health, family practice medicine, pediatrics, internal medicine, herbal medicine, acupuncture, general dentistry and nutrition, and exercise counseling. The patients who visit Min An have the opportunity to view their health and illness from both these perspectives. They may choose their therapies from either or both traditions.

In addition to the fellows of the Institute, there were members of the Institute's Board of Directors, Board of Advisers, and members of our network who played an important part in this project. Their assistance enhanced the quality of our work and they are: Jane Lurie, Charlotte Calhoun, Professor James Cahill, Dr. Stella Ling, Dr. Jerome Steiner, Dr. May Tung, Dr. Thomas Killip, and many other health professionals at major medical centers in the United States. While most of the final copies of the manuscripts were typed in China, there were many drafts that were prepared here at the Institute. We are deeply appreciative of the assistance of Dr. Wayne Payne, Judith Peck, and Faith Tan.

It was a great experience for us to work with Susan Koscielniak, Executive Editor, Columbia University Press. Ms. Koscielniak understood the vision that we had for this book. She was willing to undertake this innovative project and help us in every step of the way. We are very impressed with her insight and her publishing skills.

These bright and talented scholars in China and the United States have used their sophisticated skills and creative powers to communicate the concepts and practices of traditional Chinese medicine to the West. The effort took over six years and involved the cooperation of over twenty-four scholars to realize *The Essential Book of Traditional Chinese Medicine.*

Hanmin Liu   Dong Mianguo
President   President
United States–China Educational   People's Medical Publishing
   Institute   House
December 1986   December 1986

THE ESSENTIAL BOOK OF TRADITIONAL CHINESE MEDICINE
VOLUME 1: THEORY

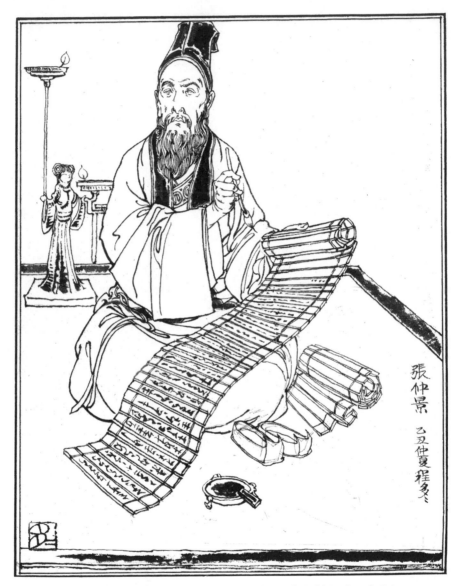

Doctor Zhang Zhongjing writing *Discussion of Cold-Induced Diseases* on bamboo.

CHAPTER ONE

———✦———

Traditional Chinese Medicine:
An Orientation

TRADITIONAL CHINESE MEDICINE is an ancient medicine, Asian in character. It views the human body as an integrated whole. Inseparable from the rest of nature, the body is defined as in opposition to nature and yet unified with it.

Such a view has grown out of millennia of study of the inner connections in the human body and of the relationship between these internal connections and the external environment.

With a cultural tradition of nearly five thousand years, China was the first to accumulate a wealth of knowledge about health and medicine. Legends show that, even in antiquity, the ancestors of today's Chinese people had already set about the task of summing up human knowledge of physiology and pathology, of the body's internal organs and channels, of etiology, diagnosis, and the principles of treatment.

For example, there are legends of *"Fu Xi* (4000 B.C.) making nine kinds of needles,"[1] an early reference to acupuncture. *Shen Nong* is a legendary character who is said to have tasted hundreds of medicinal herbs.[2] There is also the story of "the discussion of channels by Huang

1. Fu Xi, also called Fuxishi, actually denotes the time of "Fuxishi," a legendary period of primitive clan society in the history of China. According to legend, this was the time when the therapies of acupuncture and moxibustion were first invented.

2. According to the legend, Shen Nong was also known as Shennongshi (3000 B.C.), the originator of agriculture, medicine, and pharmacy. Actually, the word denotes the Shen Nong period of primitive clan society in the history of China. According to the ancient book, *Master of Huainan,* by Liu An of the Han dynasty, "Shen Nong tasted a hundred herbs and came across seventy poisonous herbs each day."

Di and Qi Bo,"[3] who are reknowned for their contributions to traditional Chinese medicine.

Today, more than 6,000 texts record the long history of clinical experience of Chinese physicians and their theoretical work in the field of medicine. As early as the Warring States period (475–221 B.C.), a monumental work of medicine appeared in China, the *Classic of Internal Medicine*.[4] It consisted of two books: the first was called *Plain Questions;* the second, *Miraculous Pivot*. Together, these volumes summarized the medical achievements of ancient China. Building on the theories of *yin-yang* and the five elements,[5] they systematically interpreted the physiology and pathology of the internal organs and the channels of the body. They recorded ancient anatomic knowledge

3. Legend has it that Huangdi was an ancient emperor in China (the Yellow Emperor of about 2695–2589 B.C.). Qi Bo was a famous physician of that period. The Emperor asked Qi Bo to taste various kinds of herbs and to study medicine and pharmacy. The first and greatest medical work in China, *Classic of Internal Medicine,* was written in the style of questions and answers between Huangdi and Qi Bo on problems of medicine and pharmacy.

4. The *Classic of Internal Medicine* is the oldest and greatest medical classic of China. Its authorship is traditionally ascribed to the ancient Emperor Huangdi. Actually, the work was a product of various unknown authors during the Warring States period. The book consists of two parts: *Plain Questions* and *Miraculous Pivot*.

Plain Questions originally consisted of nine volumes with eighty-one essays. The book addresses a variety of subjects, such as human anatomy, physiology, etiology, pathology, diagnosis, the differentiation of symptom-complexes, prevention and treatment of disease, ways to keep fit, the relationship between man and nature, the application of the theories of *yin* and *yang* and the five elements in medicine, and the theory of the promotion of the flow of *qi*.

The subjects of *Miraculous Pivot* are similar to those of *Plain Questions,* but *Miraculous Pivot* has a more detailed description of the channels and collaterals, acupuncture, and moxibustion, so it is also known as the *Canon of Acupuncture*. In introducing basic theories and clinical practice, the two books complement each other.

From this beginning, there evolved in China a literature of medicine that continuously incorporated new experience into the traditional theoretical framework. Some of the key works include *A Classic of Acupuncture and Moxibustion,* by Huangfu Mi, which was written about 259 A.D. It was based on the *Miraculous Pivot,* and further developed the theory of channels and collaterals. *The Pulse Classic,* by Wang Shuhe, further summarized and explained the 24 pulse conditions and the diseases associated with them. It contributed to systematizing the theory and methods later described in *"The General Treatise on Etiology and Symptoms of Diseases,"* by Chao Yuanfang, which was written in A.D. 610. It recorded causes and symptoms of different kinds of diseases in detail, extending the theory of etiology and pathogenesis in Chinese medicine.

5. The theory of the five elements is also known as the theory of the five phases. "Phase" is actually a more accurate translation of the Chinese "xing." Also, "phase" may be more appropriate since the theory of the five elements is a theory of change and movement, which the word "phase" implies. However, since this theory is widely known as the five elements theory, this book will also use this translation.

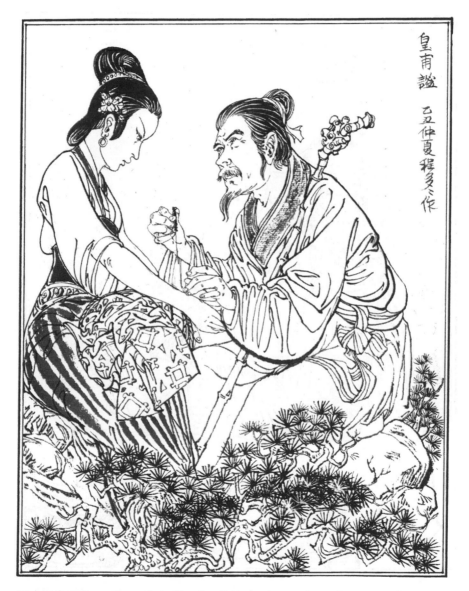

Huangfu Mi, author of *A Classic of Acupuncture*, inserting an acupuncture needle.

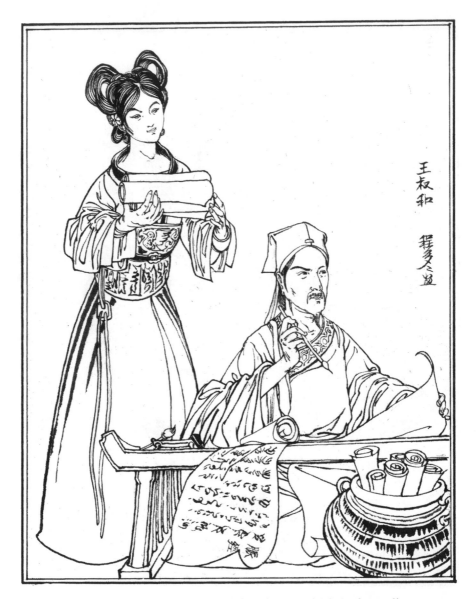

Doctor Wang Shuhe writing *The Pulse Classic*, which is the earliest comprehensive work dealing with several kinds of pulses and their diagnostic value.

of the human body: the length of various bones and vessels and the sizes and volumes of the internal organs. They introduced the idea that "the heart is the center of blood circulation and of the system of blood vessels of the human body,"[6] and that the blood circulating in vessels "is similar to a flow of water, traveling around without end."[7] The *Classic of Internal Medicine* set forth the origin of illness and defined the principles for its diagnosis and treatment. In short, it laid the foundation for the theory of traditional Chinese medicine.

In the period of the late Eastern Han dynasty (206 B.C.–A.D. 220), a second major work appeared, summarizing the experience of Chinese practitioners in the prevention and treatment of disease. This was the *Discussion of Cold-Induced Diseases.*[8]

The *Discussion of Cold-Induced Diseases* explained certain infectious diseases by describing the functioning of the major channels of the body; it also described the development of a wide range of other diseases according to the theory of the internal, or *zang-fu* organs.[9]

6. "Treatise on the Feebleness of Limbs" in *Plain Questions*.

7. "Treatise on the Length of Vessels," in *Miraculous Pivot*.

8. *Discussion of Cold-Induced Diseases and Synopsis of the Golden Chamber* were originally a single work entitled *Discussion of Cold-Induced and Miscellaneous Diseases*. Together, they summed up the experience and understanding of diagnosis and treatment that has since led to various schools of medicine. For example, the school of thought that developed in the Jin and Yuan dynasties and explained pathogenesis in terms of pathogenic fire and heat was elaborated by Liu Wansu (A.D. 1120–1200); Zhang Zihe (A.D. 1156–1228) established a theory of the conquest of pathogenic factors; Zhang Jiegu described the mechanism of disease in the *zang-fu* organs; Li Dongyuan (A.D. 1187–1251) developed a theory of the spleen and stomach; and Zhu Danxi (A.D. 1281–1358) explained the doctrine of nourishing *yin*. Works by the distinguished physicians Zhang Jingyue (A.D. 1563–1640) and Zhao Xianke (in the period of the Ming dynasty, A.D. 1368–1644) were a thorough exposition and development of the theories of *yin* and *yang*, the vital gate (the source of heat energy of the body; it is also the *yang* of the kidney, or the place where the inborn original vital energy is stored), and the relationship between the spleen and the kidney.

With the accumulation of experience in the diagnosis and treatment of febrile disease by the time of the Qing dynasty (A.D. 1644–1911), there was a breakthrough in the theory of differentiating symptom-complexes that led to a new school of heat-induced disease, represented by the well-known physicians Ye Tianshi (A.D. 1667–1746), Wu Jutong (A.D. 1758–1836), and Wang Mengying (A.D. 1808–1866). They studied the onset and development of acute infectious disease and initiated a new method for differentiating symptom-complexes according to the condition of the *"ying, qi, wei,* and *xue"* systems and the Triple Burner. (See chapter 8 for a detailed description of these methods.)

9. The Chinese describe human anatomy in terms of the *zang* and *fu* organs. These include most of the internal organs of Western medicine, but also include other structures of the body. They are divided into two classes, *zang* and *fu*. The theory of the *zang-fu* organs is the subject of chapter 3.

These descriptions later developed into a complete theory for the differentiation of symptom-complexes—the basis for diagnosis in traditional Chinese medicine.

Building on the *Classic of Internal Medicine,* the *Discussion of Cold-Induced Diseases* provided guidelines for treatment. It listed 113 prescriptions and 397 therapies for infectious diseases, as well as 265 prescriptions for miscellaneous diseases.

During the same period, the first materia medica also appeared in China. It was known as *Shen Nong's Herbal.* The ancient people of China had discovered that certain plants, animals, and mineral products could cure certain diseases. After long and repeated trials, they accumulated, step by step, reliable experience in the use of these medications. The *Herbal* is a summation of this experience and the general knowledge of pharmacy prior to the Han dynasty. It records 365 kinds of plant, animal, and mineral drugs, listing their properties and effects. Included among its prescriptions are *Rhizoma Coptis* (Chinese goldthread) for dysentery; *Radix Dichroae* (root of Dichroa) for malaria; *Herba Ephedrae* (Chinese ephedra) for asthma; *Sargassum* (kelp) for goiter; *Radix et Rhizoma Rhei* (root and rhizome of rhubarb) for constipation; and mercury for scabies. Each of these is still of clinical significance today.

Much later, during the Ming dynasty (A.D. 1368–1644), the *Herbal* was updated by Li Shizhen. As a physician and pharmacologist, Li systematized the folk experience of the previous generations by conducting his own collection and investigation of medical specimens. His book, entitled *Compendium of Materia Medica* described 1,892 medicinal substances and included over 10,000 prescriptions as well as more than 1,000 illustrations of medicinal specimens. Li's work also revised the conventional classification of medicinal substances, laying the foundation for a systematic botany. Soon after its publication, the *Compendium* was translated into several languages and gradually distributed around the world; it has achieved worldwide recognition as a major contribution to the development of medicine and systematic botany.

Many other works have recorded Chinese knowledge of substances with medicinal properties.[10] One such work, *Newly Revised Materia*

10. For example, Zhao Xuemin, a physician and pharmacologist in the Qing dynasty, expanded the *Compendium* in a book entitled *A Supplement to the Compendium of Materia Medica;* this supplement added 716 new drugs to the original.

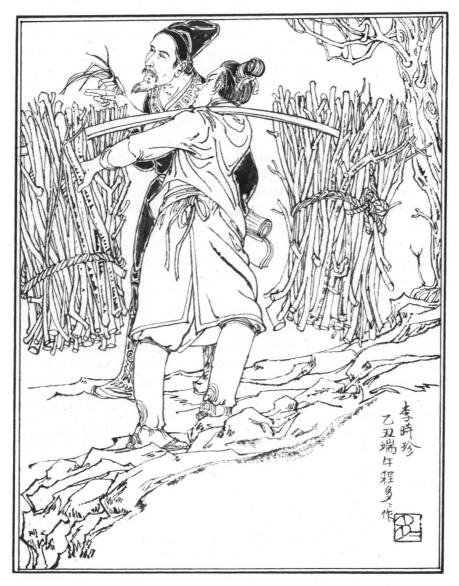

Doctor Li Shizhen, author of the *Compendium of Materia Medica,* identifying herbs.

Medica,[11] was published by the Tang dynasty government in A.D.
659 to regulate the use of drugs. Other works developed the science
of prescription.[12] Through clinical practice, the Chinese people had
begun to understand that the compound prescription, composed of
several ingredients, could enhance the curative effects of individual
ingredients and reduce the toxic effects of some drugs. Thousands of
recipes were tested and collected, and the theory of the "principal,
adjuvant, auxiliary, and conductant ingredients" gradually emerged.
This theory, together with the *Seven Kinds of Prescription Compositions*
and the *Ten Prescription Effects,* has become an important part of the
"principles, rules, prescriptions, and medications" of medical science
in China.

In addition to herbs and drugs, traditional Chinese medicine has
evolved other therapies to treat disease. Best known perhaps is acupuncture. This therapy continues to be developed today. In particular, its recent applications in anesthesiology have aroused worldwide
interest. There are also other therapies that have a folk character but
that continue to play a role in modern medical practice in China:
these include cupping; *guasha* (popular treatment by scraping); ad-
hesive plasters and the use of hot compresses; fuming or steaming,
therapies that use water, mud, wax, or magnets; massage techniques
of bonesetting; chiropractic; cutting; *qigong* (a breathing exercise
therapy); and physical exercise.

All of these are part of traditional Chinese medicine. The core of
this tradition, however, is a set of theories about the functioning of
the body and its relationship to the world around it. And at the core

11. *Newly Revised Materia Medica.* This work was compiled by a staff of twenty-two
scholars and physicians appointed by the Tang Emperor Gao Zong, and published in A.D.
659. A total of 844 medicinal substances were included.

12. The representative works are:

Prescriptions Worth a Thousand Gold and the *Supplement to the Prescriptions Worth a Thousand
Gold,* by Sun Simiao, written during the Tang dynasty (A.D. 618–907). It recorded the
achievements of tested prescriptions and clinical experience with them up to that time.

Peaceful Holy Benevolent Prescriptions, by Wang Huaiyin, written during the Song dynasty
(A.D. 960–992). This is an extensive collection of recipes developed prior to the Song
dynasty, together with folk remedies of that period. It included 16,834 prescriptions and
discussed these in relation to symptom-complexes and pathological mechanisms.

Universal Prescriptions, by Zhu Su et al., published in 1406. It contains 61,739 prescriptions and 239 illustrations of medical plants, epitomizing the essence of Chinese knowledge
of prescriptions up to the time of the Ming dynasty.

of this set of theories is one very important concept—that of integrity.

THE CONCEPT OF INTEGRITY

The concept of integrity emerges from the theory of *yin* and *yang*. This theory pervades all of Chinese science. According to it, any object in nature is both a unified whole and a whole composed of two parts with opposing qualities. These opposing qualities are described as *yin* and *yang*.

Chinese medicine views the relationship between the human being and nature as an integrated one. The human being and nature represent opposing parts of a unified integrity. At the same time, the human body is a miniature version of this enormous system—a miniature universe. Each person thus represents a unity of opposing parts.

Traditional Chinese medicine has a way of thinking called "one dividing into two." The human body can be divided into two without end—into pairs of opposing forces, functions, or parts. Examples of these pairs that are particularly important for understanding physiology and pathology, diagnosis and treatment, are: exterior and interior; upper and lower; ascending and descending; *qi* [13] and blood; essence and spirit; and *zang* organs and *fu* organs. These pairs, in opposition to each other, each explain the functioning of the whole organism. If one pair were separated from the whole, it would no longer possess its original functional properties.

Guided by the concept of integrity, traditional Chinese medicine has outlined a unique system of physiology and anatomy. It has also developed a unique approach to the practice of medicine: because the body is an integrated system, the condition of any of its parts reflects, to a certain extent, the condition of the whole. By observing the outward or "local" changes in the body—for example, observing the color of the complexion, the tongue, and the ears, or by feeling the pulse—the practitioner can judge the condition of the whole.

13. *Qi* is the activity of life. It is both the functioning of the body and a rarefied substance that actuates the body's functions. For a more complete discussion of *qi* in its many forms, see chapter 3.

The whole can be treated. This concept of integrity thus defines an approach to both diagnosis and treatment.

INTEGRITY IN THE HUMAN BODY

Traditional Chinese medicine holds that the human body is composed of various organs and tissues, each of which has its own distinct physiological function, which, in turn, is a part of the whole life activity. Because they are part of a unified whole, these organs and their physiological functions are bound to be physiologically interrelated; they are also mutually influenced by any disorder or pathology.

At the center of this organic integrity are five *zang* organs. All physiological functions begin with these five organs and are communicated throughout the body by an elaborate system of channels. Physiology in Western medicine is described in terms of the systems of circulation, respiration, digestion, reproduction, and endocrine functions. Traditional Chinese medicine, by contrast, describes five systems of physiological activity. These systems correspond to the five *zang* organs: heart, kidney, liver, lungs, and spleen.

The *zang* and *fu* organs work together in pairs, regulating each other. For example, the liver and the gallbladder constitute a pair. Furthermore, each pair of *zang-fu* organs is also related to other parts of the body: the skin, flesh, vessels, tendons, and bones, which are known as "the five tissues" in Chinese medicine. Again as an example, the tendons are considered to be most closely related to the liver-gallbladder.

The five sense organs—mouth, nose, tongue, eyes, and ears—are also related to the pairs of *zang-fu* organs; the eyes, for example, are the sense organs associated with the liver.

Finally, there are outward or superficial manifestations for each pair of *zang-fu* organs; the nails are the outward manifestation of the liver-gallbladder pair. This set of relationships is shown in figure 1.1.

The relationship between the liver and the gallbladder is one of opposition between the interior and exterior. The liver is an *interior* organ while the gallbladder is an *exterior* organ.

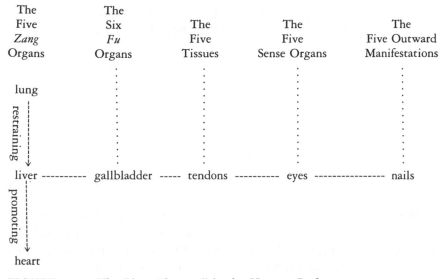

FIGURE 1.1. The Liver "System" in the Human Body

The liver is also related to the other *zang* organs. Another basic theory of Chinese science, the theory of the five elements, explains the nature of these relationships. The five elements are wood, fire, earth, metal, and water. These elements each have different qualities. The theory of the five elements thus describes the relationship among objects or phenomena of different qualities. And so it is with *zang* organs.

For example, according to traditional Chinese medicine, the liver corresponds to wood, the heart to fire, and the lungs to metal. This set of correspondences defines a set of relationships among these three organs. Since wood can feed fire, the liver is seen as promoting the functioning of the heart. The lung (metal) is seen as restraining or suppressing the functioning of the liver. In this way, the functional activities of every *zang* organ are promoted or restrained by another *zang* organ or, more properly, a *zang-fu* organ system. From this view of the body as an integrity, the individual physiological functions typically treated in Western medicine—water and food intake, digestion, absorption, conveyance, and excretion—result from the harmonious functioning of the *zang-fu* organs.

INTEGRITY IN THE RELATIONSHIP
BETWEEN HUMAN AND ENVIRONMENT

Man lives on the *qi* of heaven and earth; he grows according to the laws
of seasonal changes.

"Treatise on How to Keep Healthy"
in *Plain Questions*

Heaven feeds man with five smells: a foul smell, a scorched smell, a sweet
smell, a fishy smell, and a putrid smell. Earth feeds man with five tastes:
sour, bitter, sweet, pungent, and salty.

"Treatise on the Organ Picture"
in *Plain Questions*

Not only is the human body an organic whole, but there also
exists a relationship of integrity between the human body and nature. As long as humans live in nature, the natural environment will
determine the necessities for their existence. Any changes in the natural environment will directly or indirectly influence the human body
through its sense organs. These sense organs communicate the natural variations in the environment to the core of the human system—
to the *zang-fu* organs. As a result, physiology is not a static system,
and pathology is not a static condition. Rather, both are constantly
changing, and any treatment must recognize these changes.

That "man lives on the *qi* of heaven and earth" can be understood
more or less literally. The *"qi* of heaven and earth" implies those
substances such as air and food supplied by nature to support the life
process. That the human body "develops according to the laws of
seasonal changes" means that the body spontaneously regulates its
internal functions to adapt to the regular changes that occur in the
environment.

These statements can also be viewed, however, as symbolic statements about the relationship between the human body and the environment. Symbolically, they suggest that human physiology depends on the qualities of the environment. These are of two types,
represented by heaven and earth. To understand the dynamic nature
of the body, one must understand these qualities and how they are
reflected in the body. Also, the laws of seasonal changes denote regularities in the process of change. These regularities, too, must be
understood in order to describe human physiology at any point in
time.

When *Plain Questions* states that "heaven feeds man with five smells and earth feeds man with five tastes," it is describing qualities of the environment that are transmitted to the body. These qualities correspond to the five elements and *represent* a series of laws about the relationship between the human being and the environment in its different stages. They may also be given a literal interpretation: the five smells generally denote the quality of the air taken in, and the five tastes denote the quality of the food consumed.

Seasonal changes are thus communicated to the body through *qi* (or air) and food. Different seasons have different qualities of *qi* and food, which are described by the theory of the five elements. The seasons thus have a natural relationship with the *zang* organs, which also correspond to the five elements. Certain seasons (or climates) will nourish and promote certain *zang* organs. The liver, for example, is said to "communicate with" spring; the heart, with summer; the lung, with autumn; the kidney, with winter; and the spleen, with "late summer" (the sixth month in the lunar calendar).

These laws imply a need for adjustments in the relationship between body and environment. Under natural climatic influences, the human body must constantly adjust its physiological activities. The nature of the adjustments is as follows:

> It is a general law that generation occurs in spring, growth in summer, contraction in autumn, and storage in winter; man acts correspondingly.
> "Treatise on the Variations of Qi During the
> Day" in *Miraculous Pivot*

The mechanism of these adjustments is the body fluid. Body fluid, according to traditional Chinese medicine, emerges from the combination of the *qi,* or energy of the five *zang* organs, with the essence of the food taken in. Body fluid is thus a mirror of the environmental conditions in which the body is functioning. At the same time, the body fluids regulate the *yin* and *yang* condition of the body as well as the action of *qi* and blood in accordance with the changes of the season:

> Hot days or the wearing of a heavy coat causes the texture and interstitial spaces of the muscles to open; perspiration then occurs. On cold days, the texture and interstitial spaces of the muscles are closed, preventing

TABLE 1.1.   **Effect of Climatic Changes on the Human Body**

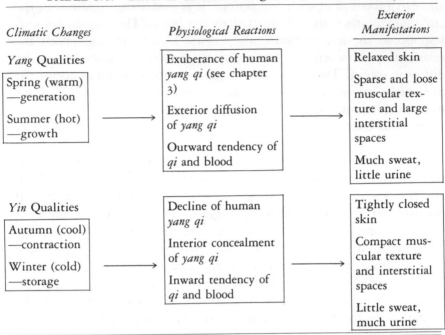

Climatic Changes	Physiological Reactions	Exterior Manifestations
Yang Qualities Spring (warm) —generation Summer (hot) —growth	Exuberance of human *yang qi* (see chapter 3) Exterior diffusion of *yang qi* Outward tendency of *qi* and blood	Relaxed skin Sparse and loose muscular texture and large interstitial spaces Much sweat, little urine
Yin Qualities Autumn (cool) —contraction Winter (cold) —storage	Decline of human *yang qi* Interior concealment of *yang qi* Inward tendency of *qi* and blood	Tightly closed skin Compact muscular texture and interstitial spaces Little sweat, much urine

the release of *qi* and moisture; in this case the water in the body flows downward, becoming urine.

"Special Treatise on the Five Disorders of the
Body Fluid" in Miraculous Pivot

The necessary adjustments between the body and environment with seasonal changes is summarized in table 1.1.

In addition to season changes, Chinese medicine contends that changes in the time of the day affect human physiological functioning. The balance between *yin* and *yang* and the behavior of *qi* and *blood* correspond to changes between day and night, dawn and dusk:

> In the daytime, the human's *yang qi* is expanding; it begins its expansion at dawn and flourishes at midday, while at sunset, it declines, and the *qi* door closes.

"Treatise on Communication of Vitality with
Heaven" in Plain Questions

The "*qi* door" refers to the body's pores, which are also called the "mysterious house"; they are the main pathway for the dispersion of body heat. (Respiration and excretion are also ways to disperse heat, but the area they cover and the amount of heat they dissipate are not as great as that of the skin.) In Western terms, *yang qi* may be thought of as heat energy, which emerges in the morning, becomes most vigorous at noon, and drops at night so as to permit the body to rest and refresh itself. So it is said in traditional Chinese medicine that "one falls asleep when *yang* enters into *yin.*"

Geographic differences shape human physiology in the same way as seasonal and diurnal conditions.

PATHOLOGY: WHEN THE BALANCE IS THREATENED

Wind, rain, cold, and heat alone can hurt no man without weak points.
"Treatise on the Primary Occurrence of
Diseases" in *Miraculous Pivot*

The point where pathogenic factors invade the body is bound to be a point where *qi* is deficient.
"Treatise on Fevers" in *Plain Questions*

If the human body and the environment are viewed as an integrated system—in which the body is constantly changing to maintain a dynamic balance with the environment—it becomes clear that disease occurs when the body is unable to maintain the balance, when it fails to adapt (see figure 1.2.).

Similarly, if the body itself is an integrated whole, then any imbalance in its internal systems is a possible source of illness.

Accordingly, traditional Chinese medicine speaks of two types of "pathogenic factors" or causes of disease. These are *exogenous* pathogenic factors, or those that come from the external environment, and *endogenous* pathogenic factors, which arise from a serious internal imbalance.

The principal exogenous factors are extreme climatic conditions: wind, cold, heat, dampness, dryness, and fire.

For example, a patient may suffer from an illness caused by "exogenous wind-cold." Exposure of the body surface to wind and cold may have created an imbalance between the defensive energy system of skin, and the muscles and interstitial spaces between the muscles. As a result, the body's resistance is lowered, and a set of symptoms perhaps including aversion to cold, fever, and a floating pulse, ap-

Exogenous Pathogenic Factors

Physical Pathogenic Factors   or   Biological Pathogens
(abnormal climatic changes)   (bacteria and viruses)

Encounter
Body Deficiency of Essential *Qi**

And Produce:
• Lower Physiological Functioning
• Decreased Adaptability
• Inability To Accommodate
• Decreased Body Resistance

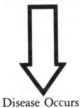

Disease Occurs

*See chapter 3.

FIGURE 1.2.   The Occurrence of Disease

pears. Since the skin is in an interior-exterior relationship with the lungs, this imbalance may affect the lungs. The functioning of the lung *qi* (see chapter 3) is reduced, and the lung fails in its normal function of dispersing the body's *qi* downward. As a result, *qi* is forced in an abnormal upward path, and a cough occurs.

However, a cough may occur not only as a result of the exogenous pathogenic factors just described, but also as the result of endogenous pathological changes in other *zang* organs that affect the lung. For example, an exuberant liver fire may be said to "flare up" and "burn" the lung, causing a cough or even the coughing up of blood. Another example of the relationship between *zang* organs is hepatitis. According to Chinese medicine the onset of this disease is due to a condition that can be described as "damp-heat" in the liver and gallbladder. Or it may be due to a depressing of the liver in which there is a stagnation of *qi*. Clinical symptoms may include nausea, vomiting, distension of the stomach and abdomen, diarrhea, and loose (shapeless) stools. These symptoms are primarily functional problems of the spleen and stomach. Chinese medicine explains that liver disorders directly affect the functioning of the spleen and stomach:

> When we discover that the liver is ill, and we know that liver disorders are readily transmitted to the spleen, the latter should be strengthened and nourished first.
>
> *Synopsis of the Golden Chamber*

Illness that originates in the internal organs of the body will also systematically affect the tissues on the body surface. Excessive liver heat may cause a flushed face and bloodshot eyes. Too much "fire" in the heart will show up as ulcers, pain, or redness of the tongue. Preponderant lung heat may induce dryness of the nose. Paleness of the lips and tongue as well as loss of appetite reveals a deficient spleen. A weakening kidney may bring about deafness or severe tinnitus.

It is clear from these relationships that in traditional Chinese medicine, pathology is not an isolated affliction of one part of the body or another. Rather it is an imbalance in the many opposing processes that make up the whole integrated organism. Not surprisingly, this view of pathology leads to an integrated approach to diagnosis and treatment as well.

DIAGNOSIS: FINDING THE PRINCIPAL IMBALANCE

> Anything inside is bound to manifest outwardly. Outward manifestations and their locality may reveal the condition of the internal organs; in this way, the location of the illness will be known.
>
> "Treatise on the Original Organs" in
> *Miraculous Pivot*

A basic principle of traditional Chinese medicine is that "anything inside is bound to manifest outwardly." This principle stems from the concept of integrity and has two important implications for diagnosis.

The first is that it is never adequate to diagnose the condition solely as a local disturbance. Local problems—such as headaches, skin rashes, and a host of other obvious symptoms—reveal functional abnormalities of certain internal organs and of the body's channel system.

For example, the sudden onset of acute conjuctivitis (called "fire-eyes" in traditional Chinese medicine) is said to be due to the flaring upward of "liver-fire." It should be treated with drugs that dispel pathogenic wind and fire from the liver. The drug typically prescribed for this condition is "gentian pills for purging the liver." This diagnosis and treatment is based on the understanding that the liver is associated with the eyes and that the liver channel communicates upward through the eyes.

Another example is deafness. Chinese medicine would say that deafness is a local symptom. Since the ears are the sense organs associated with the kidney, certain types of deafness may be diagnosed as a deficiency in the kidney; they are therefore treated by tonification of the kidney.

The second implication of the idea that "anything inside is bound to manifest outwardly" is that external symptoms, if properly analyzed, can reveal the essential nature of the illness—the essential imbalance in the system. This essential imbalance is summarized in Chinese medicine by the so-called "symptom-complex." The fundamental task of diagnosis is to differentiate among symptom-complexes.

Chinese medicine does not distinguish different *diseases;* it differentiates *symptom-complexes.* A "symptom-complex" is different from a symptom. Symptoms are manifestations such as headaches, coughing, or vomiting. A symptom-complex is a complete summarization of the functioning of the body at a particular stage of the illness. It includes symptoms, but also links these symptoms to a basic imbalance in the functioning of the body. It is possible to call the symptom-complex a *complete* summarization of the functioning of the body because, according to Chinese medicine, pathogenic factors are bound to act on an individual body in a certain way, no matter how complex they may be. There is a limit to the structure and function of the body; hence, there is also a limit to the typical conditions which pathogenic factors produce in the body.

In diagnosing illness, then, Chinese medicine does not begin with clinical symptoms, but rather with a prescribed set of observations—

observations that are guided by the theoretical distinctions between opposing parts of the body. For example, the so-called "Eight Guiding Principles" are the basis for much of the differentiation. The Eight Guiding Principles describe four opposing pairs: exterior and interior, heat and cold, deficiency and excess, *yin* and *yang*. By making observations from this point of view, the practitioner of traditional Chinese medicine can differentiate a single symptom-complex which represents the present functional condition of the body.

For example, the clinical symptoms of fever, chills, headache, or generalized aches may be related to a "cold" condition of the "exterior" or superficial region of the body. This condition is the common cold. However, the entire set of clinical observations may reveal one of two different symptom-complexes, depending on the pathogenic factors involved. One complex will result from "wind-cold," the other from "wind-heat."

The proper treatment cannot be selected unless the proper symptom-complex is identified. A superficial cold due to wind-cold would require the method known as "dispelling pathogenic factors from the exterior of the body with pungent sudorifics of a warm nature." A cold with a symptom-complex of wind-heat, on the other hand, is treated by the method known as "dispelling pathogenic factors from the exterior of the body with pungent sudorifics of a cool nature."

When diagnosis is based on differentiating symptom-complexes, several different symptom-complexes may account for a condition that, in Western medicine, is viewed as a single disease. On the other hand, the same symptom-complex can appear in a variety of different diseases at some stage in their development. Since treatment follows diagnosis, a single disease such as the common cold described above may be treated by different methods, and different diseases may be treated by the same method.

TREATMENT: RESTORING THE BALANCE

Treatment is determined by carefully looking into the relationship of *yin* and *yang* and regulating this relationship to bring them into balance.
"General Treatise on Essential Principles" in
Plain Questions

The goal of treatment in traditional Chinese medicine is to restore the balance between parts of the body and between the body and its environment. Since this balance is a dynamic one—that is, since it is constantly changing—treatment must constantly be adapted and adjusted to suit the situation. The differentiation of symptom-complexes guides this process. And as suggested above, it leads to two maxims of traditional Chinese medicine.

The first is: *Apply different methods of treatment to the same disease.* Different methods of treatment are necessary for the same disease because the symptom-complex will differ depending on when and where the disease occurs, the individual response to the pathogenic factor, and the stage of advance of the disease. For example, treatments for colds occurring in different seasons are not the same. Those caught in winter are usually caused by wind-cold and should be treated with pungent drugs that are warm in nature. Colds caught in the spring are likely to be caused by wind-heat and should be treated with pungent drugs that are cool in nature. Finally, those caught in the heat of summer are frequently caused by "damp-heat"; they should be treated with aromatic drugs that reduce turbidity to dispel heat and dampness. All of these distinctions are revealed by the process of differentiating symptom-complexes.

The second maxim is: *Treat different diseases with the same method.* It may be appropriate to apply the same method of treatment to different kinds of diseases since, at any given stage, different diseases may have the same symptom-complex. For example, protracted dysentery and prolapse of the rectum or uterus are different diseases. But they are all marked by the symptom-complex of "sinking of middle *qi.*" The appropriate treatment in each case is the "lifting of middle *qi.*" Similarly, diseases such as cardiopathy (including coronary or rheumatic heart disease), nephritis, and asthma may all, at some stage in their development, show symptoms of distress in the lumbar region, weakness of the legs and a sensation of cold and chills. If such symptoms are present, those diseases can all be classified as belonging to the symptom-complex of "deficiency of kidney *yang.*"

Differentiating symptom-complexes also allows the practitioner to adjust treatment to climatic and seasonal conditions, to geographical localities, and to the patient's constitution. For example, in selecting medicines, the practitioner must work in harmony with environmental factors. In summer, when the muscular texture is loose and perspiration occurs readily, it is inappropriate to use diaphoretic drugs that are pungent in flavor and warm, dry, or hot in nature; to do so might cause excess sweating which would lead to the consumption of body fluid. In the cold of winter, when the muscular texture is contracted, *yang qi* or active energy is "concealed" and the body is relatively delicate. In this case, drugs with a bitter flavor and cold nature may produce preponderant cold, impairing *yang qi* and thereby creating a symptom-complex of endogenous cold.

The patient's constitution must also be considered when determining medications. For example, if a patient has a constitution of "exuberant *yang*" and an intolerance for heat, drugs of a warm or hot nature could exaggerate the imbalance between *yin* and *yang* by injuring the body's *vital* substances. If a patient has an intolerance to cold due to a constitutional deficiency of *yang,* cool or cold drugs should be rejected to avoid damage to the body's *yang qi.*

In all of these cases, the differentiating of symptom-complexes serves as a guide since the symptom-complex summarizes the whole situation—the internal imbalance and the imbalance between the body and the environment. Ultimately, treatment in Chinese medicine is the process of "carefully looking into the relationship of *yin* and *yang* and regulating this relationship to bring them into balance." The body's response to pathogenic factors will take one of two forms: hyperfunctioning or hypofunctioning. The aim of treatment is to adjust and help sustain the body's own balancing system to reestablish the normal equilibrium. For this reason, traditional Chinese medicine always works with both the positive and negative aspects of the condition. A treatment should not reduce the vital energy of the body while dispelling pathogenic factors. It should not impair *yin* while fortifying *yang.* Instead, it should reinforce the body's vital energy while dispelling pathogenic factors; it should enhance the body's resistance while reducing conditions of excess. Although the root cause of such imbalances and their mechanisms (i.e., the exonogenous and endogenous pathogenic factors themselves) may not be *directly* dealt with by traditional Chinese medicine, the concept of differentiating symptom-complexes to determine treatment makes it possible to conceptualize the basic patterns of such imbalances and to rectify or regulate them according to consistent rules so as to enable the patient to regain a state of balance.

The differentiation of symptom-complexes is thus a prerequisite for determining treatment. The treatment, in turn, is the practical test of the accuracy of the judgments made in differentiating symptom-complexes.

A SYSTEM OF THEORIES

These ideas—the concept of integrity in the body and between the body and the environment, the idea that illness is the result of imbalance, that diagnosis must identify the imbalance, and that treatment must restore the balance—are not the product of a single medical theory. Indeed, traditional Chinese medicine is not a single theory, but rather a system of theories—seven in all.

The remaining chapters of this book discuss these seven theories in detail. However, since they are all interrelated, it would be difficult to discuss one without referring to the others. For this reason, they are summarized here to provide a starting place for the discussions that follow.

The seven theories are:

THE THEORY OF *YIN-YANG* AND THE FIVE ELEMENTS. The theories of *yin-yang* and the five elements actually belong to the larger world of Chinese science. They provide a dynamic system of classification for objects, processes, and forces in nature. As already explained, the theory of *yin-yang* states that any object in nature is both a unified whole and a whole composed of two parts with opposing qualities. These opposing qualities are described as *yin* and *yang.* The first step of analysis is thus to classify the *yin* and *yang* aspects of the object or process being studied.

The theory of the five elements represents a further stage of classification. The five elements are labeled wood, fire, earth, metal, and water. These names stand for a combination of qualities that are unique to each element. Thus, when the Chinese say that the liver is like wood, they are saying that it exhibits the same set of qualities as the other members of this class—the class represented by wood. This classification system not only divides things into classes; it also describes the relationships among these classes. Just as the *yin* and *yang* components of any system are said to oppose or contradict each other, the five elements are also systematically related: the relationship is cyclical. It is based on the promotion and restraint of the qualities of each element. Thus, the qualities of wood are said to promote the qualities of fire, while the properties of metal restrain the properties of wood.

In the context of Chinese medicine, the theory of *yin-yang* leads to the study of opposites in the structure of the human body and in its physiology and pathology. The theory of the five elements defines a set of principles for diagnosis and treatment based on the relationships among the elements.

THE THEORY OF ZANG-FU ORGANS. The theory of the *zang-fu* organs defines the internal organs of the body and the energy system that links them with one another and with the rest of the body. According to this theory, there are five *zang* and six *fu* organs in the body. The five *zang* organs are the liver, heart, lung, spleen, and kidney. The six *fu* organs are the gallbladder,[14] small intestine, stomach, large intestine, bladder, and Triple Burners.[15] In addition, there are several miscellaneous organs: the brain, marrow, bones, blood vessels, gallbladder, and uterus.

The study of these organs includes the study of their physiological functions together with those of their related tissues. The theory also describes the production and transformation of essence, *qi,* blood, and body fluid. These are the products of the functional activities of the *zang-fu* organs; at the same time, they are the material basis for these functional activities. The theory of the *zang-fu* organs is an important component of the system that guides the differentiation of symptom-complexes and thus helps to determine diagnosis and treatment.

THE THEORY OF THE CHANNEL SYSTEM. The channel system is the energy network of the body. The theory of the channel system describes the physiological functions and the pathological changes

14. The gallbladder is classified both as a *fu* organ and as a miscellaneous organ. (See chapter 3.)

15. The Triple Burner refers to three parts of the body cavity: (1) The upper burner is the portion above the diaphragm; it houses the heart and the lung. (2) The middle burner is that portion of the cavity between the diaphragm and the navel; it houses the spleen and stomach. (3) The lower burner is the portion below the navel; it houses the kidney, urinary bladder, and the small and large intestines. The liver is also associated with the lower burner due to its special relationship with the kidney. (See chapter 3.)

that occur in this system; it relates these functions and changes to the *zang-fu* organs.

The channels are seen as an integrated organizational system that links the exterior and interior of the body as well as its upper and lower parts. The system also joins the various *zang-fu* organs and serves as a passageway through which *qi* and blood circulate.

This theory defines the Twelve Principal Channels and the Eight Miscellaneous Channels—their organization, distribution, and flow, as well as their relationship to each other. It also describes the path of circulation of individual channels as well as the implications of the channels for physiology and pathology, diagnosis and treatment.

THE THEORY OF ETIOLOGY. In traditional Chinese medicine, the study of etiology—the cause of disease—is the study of the factors that produce symptom-complexes. These factors, as already suggested, are of two principal types: exogenous and endogenous. Each pathogenic factor has a characteristic path of development. The study of etiology is the study of these characteristic paths: the way the various pathogenic factors interreact with the body to produce distinct symptom-complexes.

THE THEORY OF PATHOGENESIS. The causes of disease outlined by the theory of etiology are only the *conditions* under which disease occurs. The theory of pathogenesis describes the laws that govern the onset, development, and outcome of disease. According to this theory, all diseases have two causes: (1) the pathogenic factors or conditions described by the theory of etiology; and (2) the antipathogenic factor or the internal resistance of the body. Pathology is the result of the struggle between these two factors, and the nature of the struggle determines the course of the disease.

THE THEORY OF METHODS OF EXAMINATION. Traditional Chinese medicine outlines four classes of techniques for collecting clinical information about disease and for observing pathological changes. These are: (1) looking; (2) listening and smelling; (3) asking; and (4) feeling, including pulse taking. Particularly important among these are inspection of the tongue and pulse taking. These methods of examination are linked theoretically to the differentiation of symptom-complexes.

THE THEORY OF THE DIFFERENTIATION OF SYMPTOM-COMPLEXES. The differentiation of symptom-complexes is the fundamental method for recognizing and understanding any disease in traditional Chinese medicine. It defines the procedure for inferring a patient's condition by analyzing and synthesizing the information provided by the four methods of observation noted above. The differentiation identifies the cause, location, and nature of the disease and guides decisions about treatment. This approach to differentiation is based on an understanding of several systems for describing the body. Primary among these is the integrated system of the Eight Guiding Principles or four pairs of basic oppositions. Other systems of analysis are based on: (1) the functioning of the *zang-fu* organs; (2) the *qi,* blood, and body fluid; (3) the Six Channels; (4) a system that includes *"wei, qi, ying,* and *xue"*;[16] and (5) the functioning of Triple Burners.

One final word of orientation: these seven theories define a *qualitative* approach to understanding physiology, pathology, diagnosis, and treatment. Because they are qualitative, they make use of analogies and metaphors. In comparison to the quantitative methods of Western medicine, these analogies may seem more poetic than scientific. However, these apparently poetic classification schemes represent thousands of years of clinical observations. If their validity is compromised by the lack of statistical analysis, it is perhaps compensated for by a long and documented history.

THE RECORD OF TRADITIONAL CHINESE MEDICINE

The achievements of traditional Chinese medicine have influenced medical practice around the world. Among the "firsts" that Chinese medicine can claim are:

The Classic of Internal Medicine. This compendium was the first written presentation of a comprehensive medical theory. Its descriptions of the shape, structure, and functional changes in the organs,

---

16. *Wei, qi, ying,* and *xue* are the principal substances and energies required for maintaining the vital activities of human life. The *wei* system is the superficial defensive system of the body; the *qi* system is the secondary defensive system of the body; the *ying* system is the nutrient system; and *xue* system is the blood system. These represent successively deeper strata of the body and may be used to determine the location and seriousness of a disease.

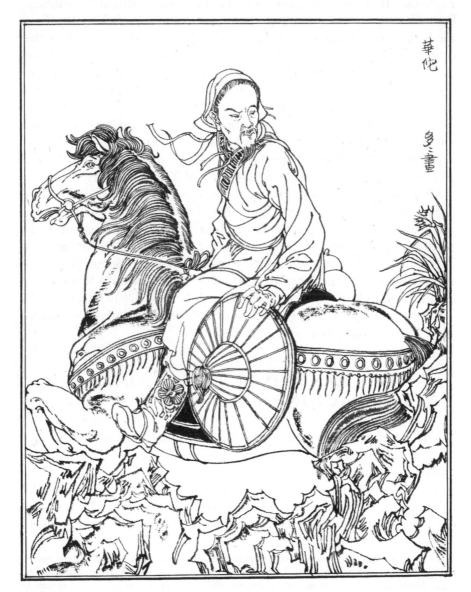

Hua Tuo, the physician who developed the remedy, "boiling anesthetic powder mixture," searching for herbs.

its conceptualization of *qi* and blood circulation in channels and vessels, and its hypotheses concerning metabolism and transformation of matter were all the most advanced at that time.

Surgery. About 1,700 years ago, Hua Tuo, a distinguished physician, invented the "Far-reaching Anesthetic Powder Mixture." Using it, he performed laparotomies and wound expansions—surgeries that were unprecedented in the world.

Preventive medicine. The Chinese system of medicine was one of the earliest to recognize the importance of preventive care and to develop techniques to avoid disease. The *Classic of Internal Medicine* commands its readers to "treat before disease arises." Also recorded were approaches to building health, cultivating moral character, and using breathing and physical exercise to keep fit. In fact, the Chinese "theory of keeping fit" is a valuable resource for the development of gerontology today. The "Frolics of Five Animals," initiated by Hua Tuo, has proven to be the pioneering approach to physical exercise therapy. Also, early in the Zhou dynasty (1066–225 B.C.), the Chinese had already learned the importance of killing rats, getting rid of rabid dogs, and other preventive measures to improve personal and environmental hygiene.

Inoculation. It was in China in the eleventh century that inoculation with a serum of human smallpox was first used as a vaccination against disease.

Pharmaceutical Chemistry. China can claim to be the first to study pharmaceutical chemistry. Ge Hong, a physician of the Jin dynasty (A.D. 320), studied "pill-making for longevity" and wrote *A Treatise on Alchemy,* which recorded the experience of the Chinese people in pharmaceutical chemistry up to that time. The book was introduced to Europe during the Sui-Tang dynasties (A.D. 581–906).

Classification of Medicine. The first relatively integrated system of medicinal classification appeared in China. Sometime in the Zhou dynasty, which spans the period from 1000 to 221 B.C., a clear classification of medicine was produced. During the Tang-Song dynasties (A.D. 618–1279), medicine was divided into such branches as diseases requiring treatment with "heavy recipes," meaning large dosages or prescriptions containing multiple ingredients, and diseases requiring treatment with "mild recipes," meaning small dosages or few ingredients, as well as gynecology, ophthalmology, stomatology,

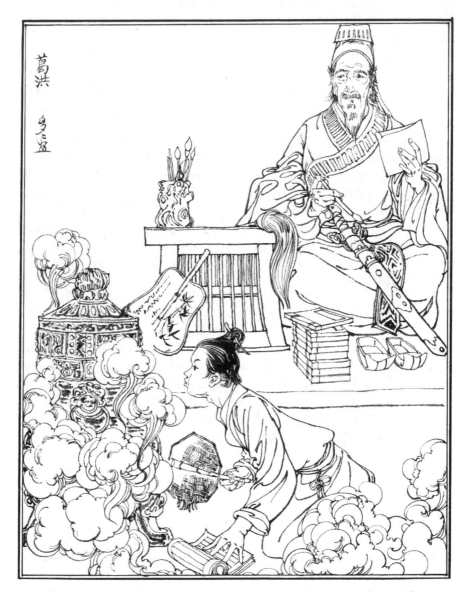

Ge Hong, the first pharmacist, overseeing the preparation of an herbal remedy, "golden pills."

laryngology, orthopedics, acupuncture, and treatment of incised wounds.

Forensic medicine. The *Instructions to Coroners,* by Song Ci, was completed in A.D. 1247. It was the earliest book in the world on forensic medicine and remains a useful reference today.

In addition to these historical contributions, traditional Chinese medicine is currently engaged in medical research that may inaugurate new methods in several areas: treating the deaf and mute with acupuncture; extracting cataracts with a technique known as snare-couching; using Chinese herbs to treat acute abdominal conditions, and to stimulate blood circulation and eliminate blood stasis; strengthening the immune system using Chinese herbs; and treatment of bone fractures using a combination of motion therapy and the fixation therapy more familiar to Western medicine.

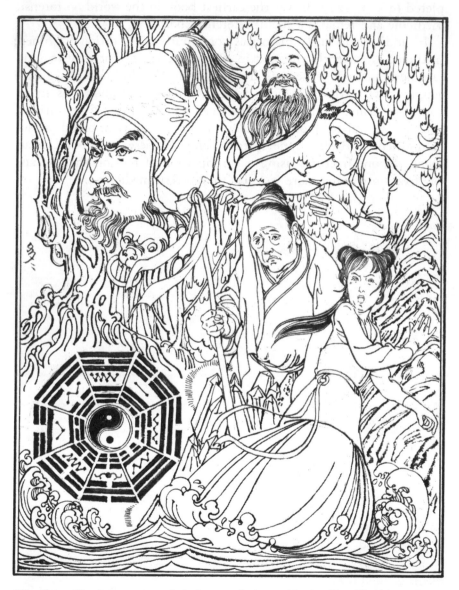

The five affective states and their correlation with the Five Elements. From top left to lower right: anger (wood), joy (fire), desire (earth), sorrow (metal), and fear (water).

CHAPTER TWO

———————◆◆◆———————

Yin-Yang
and the Five Elements

ANCIENT CHINESE SCIENCE has its roots in two philosophical systems: the theory of *yin* and *yang* and the theory of the five elements.

The early Chinese saw a material world that was constantly evolving as the result of the antagonistic movement of two opposing material forces. They called these two opposing forces *yin* and *yang*. The study of their relationship became the study of the motion and change of all things in nature.

The ancient philosophers also sought to understand the behavior of objects and phenomena in nature. They identified five fundamental elements—wood, fire, earth, metal, and water. By analogy, the characteristics and behavior of these elements further explained the principles by which natural phenomena evolved.

The theories of *yin* and *yang* and the five elements seek to explain the cause and principles of motion and change in the natural world. They have therefore been the starting point for the study of epistemology and methodology in China and have shaped the development of much academic thought. They have also become the theoretical basis for several distinct sciences. One of these is traditional Chinese medicine.

YIN–YANG AND THE UNITY OF OPPOSITES

Yin and *Yang* are the *dao*[1] of heaven and earth, the principle and plan of all things, the parents of all change, the origin of birth and death, and the source of all mysteries.

"Treatise on the Correspondence between Man
and the Universe," in *Plain Questions*

The theory of *yin* and *yang* is a dialectical system of thought: it poses two opposite forces as the underlying cause of all change. At the same time, it emphasizes the unity of these opposites.

Yin and *yang* are the general terms for the opposing aspects of objects or phenomena in nature. They may represent two opposing objects or two opposite aspects within a single object. In all situations, they are interdependent. *Yin* does not exist without *yang,* nor does *yang* exist without *yin.* In opposing each other, they create unity.

From this starting point, the ancient Chinese developed a system of thought that encompasses five basic ideas:

—All phenomena can be classified as either *yin* or *yang.*
—*Yin* and *yang* are relative concepts.
—*Yin* and *yang* are interdependent.
—The relationship between *yin* and *yang* is constantly changing.
—Under certain conditions *yin* may transform into *yang,* and *yang* into *yin.*

The theory of *yin* and *yang* explains these basic ideas as follows.

All Phenomena Can Be Classified as Either Yin or Yang.

Yin and *yang* exist in everything in nature, not only in inanimate objects, but also in living things. In each object or phenomenon, either *yin* or *yang* predominates. Accordingly, all phenomena can be classified as either *yin* or *yang.*

This classification is by no means arbitrary. Observable properties of any given object or phenomenon determine its classification. Two natural symbols guide this classification process. These are "fire" and

---

1. "Dao" may be translated as "law."

"water," which, in Chinese thought, are viewed as diametrical to each other in nature. The concrete properties of these two opposites define the abstract concepts of *yin* and *yang*. Hence, it is said that

> Water pertains to *yin,* fire pertains to *yang; qi* refers to *yang,* food refers to *yin*.
>
> "Treatise on the Correspondence Between Man
> and the Universe" in *Plain Questions*

Fire defines *yang*. Any object that has properties similar to those of fire—such as warmth, brightness, excitation, lightness, activity, or a tendency to rise—may be described as *yang*.

Water defines *yin*. Objects that tend to be cold, dim, inhibitory, heavy, and quiescent or which tend to fall or descend are classified as *yin*.

Every object in nature is either predominantly *yang* or predominantly *yin*. Every phenomenon—whether the motion of the sun, moon, and other celestial bodies; the alternating of day and night; the change of seasons; the variation of cold and heat; or even the variation in functional conditions of the body—is the result of the interplay of these two aspects.

> Heaven is *yang,* earth *yin;* the sun is *yang,* the moon *yin*.
>
> "Treatise on the Division and Junction
> of *Yin* and *Yang*" in *Plain Questions*

Thus, the heavens, being above, are *yang;* the earth, being below, is *yin*. Objects in a state of rest or quiescence are said to be *yin* or in a *yin* condition, while those that are in a state of motion are *yang*.

Yin and *yang* also define the relationship between energy and matter. The *yang* aspect of any object is that which may become vital energy. The *yin* aspect gives substance and form to an object. Thus it may be said that *qi* is *yang* and that any material form that reflects the activity of *qi* is *yin*.

Yin and Yang Are Relative Concepts.

> There is *yang* within *yin* and *yin* within *yang*. From dawn until noon, the *yang* of heaven is the *yang* within the *yang*. From noon until dusk, the *yang* of heaven is the *yin* within the *yang*. From dusk until midnight, the

yin of heaven is the *yin* within the *yin*. From midnight until dawn, the *yin* of heaven is the *yang* within the *yin*.

"Treatise on Essential Laws of Disease
Occurrence" in *Plain Questions*

While the properties associated with *yin* and *yang* are absolute, invariable, and incapable of change, the *yin* or *yang* properties of any single object in nature are not absolute and unchangeable, but relative and variable. This relativity of *yin* and *yang* has two implications. First, under certain conditions, *yin* may transform into *yang*, and *yang* may transform into *yin;* this is a basic concept in the theory of *yin* and *yang* and is described below in more detail.

Second, every object itself can be divided into two aspects: a *yin* aspect and a *yang* aspect. *Yin* can be subdivided into *yin* and *yang;* so can *yang*. Furthermore, this process can be continued indefinitely. Thus, every object or phenomenon has an infinite set of *yin* and *yang* aspects. The Chinese say "an object can be infinitely divided from one into two."

In the above quote from *Plain Questions,* the example is day and night. Day is *yang;* night is *yin*. But both may be subdivided. The morning of the day represents the *yang* part of the day. It is said to be the *yang* within the *yang*. The afternoon is the *yin* part of the day—the *yin* within the *yang*. Night can be viewed similarly. The time before midnight is the *yin* within the *yin;* between midnight and dawn is the *yang* period of the night, or the *yang* within the *yin*.

This divisibility of *yin* and *yang* is summarized as follows:

Now *yin* and *yang* can be extended from one to ten, from ten to a hundred, from a hundred to a thousand, from a thousand to ten thousand. A number as large as a thousand can hardly be counted, but the rule remains the same.

"Treatise on the Division and Junction
of *Yin* and *Yang*" in *Plain Questions*

Yin and *yang* depend on each other for existence. Without *yin,* there would be no *yang*. Without *yang,* there would be no *yin*. Neither can exist in isolation. The Chinese again point to examples from natural phenomena, such as heat and cold. Heat is *yang;* cold, *yin*. Without heat, we could not speak of cold; there would, in fact, be no cold. Without cold, there would be no heat. The same applies to the experience of "above" and "below." Without *yang* above, there would be no *yin* below; without "below" there would be no "above." This mutual dependence—or interdependence—also determines the conditions under which *yin* transforms into *yang* and *yang* into *yin*. As will be explained below, such transformation would be impossible without this interdependence.

The Relationship Between Yin and Yang Is Constantly Changing.

> The flow of *qi* pertains to *yang* and the accumulation of *qi* to *yin*. More flow means less accumulation and more accumulation means less flow. The state between flow and accumulation is constantly changing.
>
> "Illustrated Supplement to the Classic
> of Categories"

In any object or phenomenon, the opposing aspects of *yin* and *yang* are not fixed, but in a state of constant motion. The fundamental pattern of this motion is described as the interconsuming and inter-supporting of *yin* and *yang*. The consumption of *yang* leads to a supporting (or gaining) of *yin,* while the consumption of *yin* results in a supporting (or gaining) of *yang.*

For example, seasonal changes in nature illustrate the waxing and waning of *yin* and *yang*. The decrease of cold and the increase of warmth from spring to summer represent the waning (or consumption) of *yin* and the waxing (or supporting) of *yang,* while the decrease in warmth and the upsurge of cold from autumn to winter represents the waning of *yang* and waxing of *yin*. The normal seasonal interconsuming and intersupporting of *yin* and *yang* thus lead to cold, hot, warm, and cool variations in climate.

Under normal conditions, this pattern of change continues its balancing act because *yin* and *yang* restrain each other. The consumption and gaining remain within limits, so that neither *yin* nor *yang* is excessive or insufficient. *Yang* will not become excessive when it is supported by *yin.* In this way, the normal development of things is maintained.

Under abnormal conditions, however, the usual harmonious relationship of interrestraint between *yin* and *yang* is lost. Either aspect may then become excessive or insufficient. These concepts of a relative dynamic balance between *yin* and *yang* and of the possibility for excess or insufficiency of *yin* or *yang* are key concepts in traditional Chinese medicine: they explain human physiology and pathology, as well as the effect of climatic variations on the body.

Yin May Transform into Yang, and Yang into Yin.

Excessive *yin* will transform into *yang* and excessive *yang* into *yin*. Extreme cold leads to heat and extreme heat to cold.

"Treatise on the Correspondence between Man
and the Universe" in *Plain Questions*

There must be quiescence after motion, and so extreme *yang* turns into *yin*.

"Treatise on the Matching of the Circuit Phases
and Climatic Factors" in *Plain Questions*

Under certain circumstances, *yin* and *yang* within an object will transform one into the other. This transformation is the result of the basic motion of *yin* and *yang*. When the consuming/supporting relationship between *yin* and *yang* reaches a certain stage of development, *yin* may transform into *yang* and vice versa. The stages of waxing and waning of *yin* and *yang*—such as the rise and fall of temperature within a season may be viewed as stages of quantitative change in the *yin* and *yang* aspects of an object or phenomenon. The intertransformation of *yin* and *yang,* as occurs in the change of seasons, represents a *qualitative* change.

The stage at which the transformation occurs is described as "extreme." Thus *extreme* cold becomes heat. However, this extreme is relative. The exact point or condition that represents the extreme— the condition under which *yin* and *yang* transform one into the other— differs from situation to situation. Again seasonal changes provide an example. From spring to summer, the air grows warmer day by day. But when it becomes intensely hot, it then turns cooler. From autumn to winter, the air grows colder day by day. But when it reaches the extreme cold, it must again turn warmer.

Together with the previous four concepts, the idea of the intertransformation of *yin* and *yang* forms the basis for understanding the "unity of opposites" in the theory of *yin* and *yang*. All organisms, including the human body, originate from the harmony of *yin* and *yang,* which are in opposition to each other. Thus:

> *Yin* and *yang* are the origin of life.
> "Treatise on the Communication of Vitality
> with Heaven" in *Plain Questions*

THE UNITY OF OPPOSITES IN THE HUMAN BODY

> Man, because he has a form from the time of birth, depends on none
> other than *yin* and *yang.*
> "Treatise on How to Keep Healthy," in *Plain
> Questions*

The theory of *yin* and *yang,* when applied to medicine, describes the human body as an organic whole, unified but with opposing aspects. While all of the parts join together and cooperate closely with each other, they—like all phenomena in nature—can be classified according to their characteristics as either *yin* or *yang.* As with other phenomena, these classifications are relative, and a part of the body that is classified as *yang* can be further subdivided into its *yin* and *yang* aspects.

The idea of the interdependence of *yin* and *yang* also dominates traditional Chinese medicine. It is applied extensively in the understanding of physiology, pathology, and treatment. There is a common expression in traditional Chinese medicine that embodies this idea of interdependence. It is:

> Substance corresponds to *yin,* and function corresponds to *yang.*

This statement is a description of the physiology of the human body. The assertion that "substance corresponds to *yin*" means that the tangible objects of the body, such as the organs, blood, and body fluid, are all *yin* in nature. The observation that "function corresponds to *yang*" means that the transport and transformation of these substances represent the *yang* aspect of the human body. In concert with the theory of *yin* and *yang,* the body substances and their physiological activities—or functions—are mutually dependent.

The *yin* and *yang* of the human body, like the *yin* and *yang* of the universe, are constantly changing in their relationship to each other. For example, the functional *(yang)* activities of the body are bound to consume a certain amount of nutrient *(yin)* substance; this is the process of "gaining *yang* and consuming *yin.*"

Conversely, the metabolism of nutrient substances requires an expenditure of a certain amount of energy; this is the process of "gaining *yin* and consuming *yang.*" Under normal physiological conditions, the gaining and consuming of *yin* and *yang* create a state of relative dynamic balance. The process of maintaining the balance between *yin* and *yang* is the action of the human body that averts illness. Hence, the ancient Chinese wrote:

> When *yin* is even and *yang* is firm, a relative equilibrium is maintained, and health is guaranteed.
>
> "Treatise on the Communication of Vitality
> with Heaven" in *Plain Questions*

So it is that the basic ideas of the theory of *yin* and *yang*—the universality of *yin* and *yang,* their relativity, interdependence, motion, and transformation—lead to a set of ideas about the human body that, collectively, shape traditional Chinese medicine. These ideas and their roots in the theory of *yin* and *yang* may be summarized as follows.

Yin-Yang and Relativity in the Structure of the Body

> The chest cavity, lying above, corresponds to *yang,* in which the heart is the *yang* within the *yang,* while the lung is the *yin* within the *yang.* The abdominal cavity, lying below, corresponds to *yin* in which the kidney is the *yin* within the *yin* while the liver is the *yang* within the *yin* and the spleen the extreme *yin* within the *yin.*
>
> "Treatise on the Essential Laws of Disease
> Occurrence" in *Plain Questions*

All parts of the human body can be classified as either *yin* or *yang.* For example:

—The exterior of the body corresponds to *yang;* the interior, to *yin.*
—The back is *yang;* the abdomen is *yin.*
—The head is *yang;* the foot is *yin.*

These divisions into *yin* and *yang* can be further subdivided. Thus:

—The body surface, which is *yang,* can be divided into skin, which
is *yang,* and muscles and tendons, which are *yin.*
—Among the internal organs, there are six *fu* organs, which are
yang, and five *zang* organs, which are *yin.*
—Each *zang-fu* organ also has two aspects; the heart encompasses
both heart *yang* and heart *yin.*
—According to their routes, the channels can also be classified as
yin and *yang.* Those traveling along the lateral or outer side of the
extremities and across the back are *yang;* those that lie along the
medial side or inside of the extremities and that traverse the abdominal part of the body are *yin.*

These classifications are not absolute, however. They are relative.
For example, in describing the relationship between the chest and
back, Chinese medicine notes that the chest is *yin* and the back is
yang. But if the relationship between the chest and abdomen is described, the chest is no longer viewed as *yin.* In relation to the abdomen, it is *yang,* because it is above, while the abdomen, being
below, is *yin.*

Similarly, the classification of the *zang* organs changes when they
are considered in relation to each other. Thus, the heart and lung,
located in the upper trunk, are viewed as the *zang* organs that are
yang in character, while the liver, spleen, and kidney, located in the
lower trunk are seen as *yin.* Furthermore, the lung is the *yin* organ
within the *yang;* the liver is the *yang* organ within the *yin;* and the
kidney and spleen are *yin* organs within the *yin.*

In Chinese medicine, then, the *yin-yang* character of any part of
the body is a statement about its character relative to the rest of the
body. This system for characterizing the organs and tissues provides
a way of describing the complicated linkages and continuing changes
in the human body.

Yin-Yang and Body Defenses

Yin in the interior is the keeper of *yang; yang* in the exterior is the servant
of *yin.*

"Treatise on the Correspondence between Man
and the Universe" in *Plain Questions*

Yin stores essence and activates *qi; yang* defends the exterior to strengthen the body.

"Treatise on the Communication of Vitality
with Heaven" in *Plain Questions*

Chinese medicine divides physiology into two types of body functions: the defensive functions that protect the body from pathogenic factors, and the functional activities of the internal organs.

There are both *yin* and *yang* defensive functions. The *yang* defensive functions concern the exterior of the body; they provide external protection for the internal organs. The *yin* defensive functions are the interior functions; these provide the material foundation for the *yang* functions—that is, the storage and supply of body energy.

For example, when it is functioning normally, vital energy (or *yang*) produces a strong resistance on the body's surface and keeps the human body safe from attack by pathogenic factors. If pathogenic factors succeed in penetrating this superficial defense, the vital essence and blood (or *yin*) in the interior of the body will immediately respond.

Yin-Yang and the Functions of the Internal Organs

The internal organs of traditional Chinese medicine are the *zang-fu* organs. The five *zang* organs are *yin;* they control the storage of vital substances and *qi*. The six *fu* organs are *yang;* they control the transport and digestion of food. Thus, storage is a *yin* function, while the transport and transformation of substances is a *yang* function.

As indicated above, each of the *zang* and *fu* organs can be further subdivided into *yin* and *yang*. The activity or function of the organ is its *yang* aspect, while its substance is its *yin* aspect. For example, the heart is said to control the circulation of blood and mental activities; these activities constitute heart *yang*. The blood and the organ substance of the heart are heart *yin*.

In accordance with the idea that *yin* can transform into *yang* and vice versa, substance and activity in the human body can be transformed one into the other, according to traditional Chinese medicine. Substance *(yin)* produces *yang qi;* it is the material basis for *yang qi*. At the same time, substance *(yin)* is itself continually produced by the physiological action of *yang qi*. This intertransformation proceeds continuously, maintaining a relative balance in the body.

The theory of *yin* and *yang* also helps explain the *functional state* of the organs. Excitation is *yang;* inhibition is *yin*. Hyperfunctioning is a *yang* state; hypofunctioning is a *yin* state.

Yin and *yang* describe the movement of body fluid and *qi* through the body, too:

> Air *(yang)* exits from the upper openings, while wastes *(yin)* exit from the lower openings. *Yang* travels through the tissues and interstitial spaces, while *yin* travels through the five *zang* organs. *Yang* strengthens the four extremities, while *yin* acts within the six *fu* organs.
>
> "Treatise on the Correspondence between Man
> and the Universe" in *Plain Questions*

Anything light and clear or thin is thought to have a *yang* character, while anything weighty and turbid or thick is *yin*. Therefore, human *yang*—the light, clear fresh air, and food energy in the body—nourishes and strengthens the limbs; it is evaporated through the skin, tissue, interstitial spaces, and the mouth and nose to maintain their normal functioning. Human *yin*—the weighty and turbid or thick substances in the body—are transformed into food essence and stored in the five *zang* organs; wastes are eliminated via the six *fu* organs through the lower openings—the urethra and anus—to maintain the normal metabolism of food and fluid.

Pathology and the Lack of Balance

> When turbulence becomes extreme, quiescence arises to compose; when *yin* predominates, *yang* comes to control.
>
> "Principles of Medical Lore in the Book of
> Changes" in *Sub-Systematic Classic of Categories*
>
> *Yin* in excess makes *yang* suffer; *yang* in excess makes *yin* suffer. A preponderance of *yang* leads to heat manifestations; a preponderance of *yin* brings on cold.
>
> "Treatise on the Correspondence Between Man
> and the Universe" in *Plain Questions*

In a healthy body, as in the universe, the relationship between *yin* and *yang* is constantly changing. *Yin* and *yang* continuously support and consume each other. This pattern of change is known as "mutual restraint" of *yin* and *yang;* it produces a dynamic equilibrium—a balance—in the body. If this pattern of mutual restraint fails, however, the balance is lost. A preponderance or deficiency of *yin* or *yang* appears. The body is then transformed from its healthy state into a morbid one.

Traditional Chinese medicine recognizes four types of imbalance. These may be characterized as follows:

- *Yang* impaired by a preponderance of *yin*
- *Yin* consumed by a preponderance of *yang*
- An overabundance of *yang* caused by a deficiency of *yin*
- An overabundance of *yin* resulting from a deficiency of *yang*

The type of imbalance that occurs depends on the source of the imbalance. There are two sources. First are the pathogenic factors that the body encounters in nature; these are generally called "exogenous pathogenic factors." Second is a change in the body's own resistance. This resistance is sometimes called the endogenous "antipathogenic factor" or simply antipathogenic *qi.*

Both exogenous and endogenous factors may be classified as either *yin* or *yang.* The antipathogenic factor, including vital function, is *yang,* while vital essence is *yin.* Furthermore, the two are interrelated. Any excess or deficiency of the *yin* or *yang* of either the pathogenic or antipathogenic factors will influence the other. In general, exogenous pathogenic factors tend to produce conditions of excess— that is, a preponderance of either *yin* or *yang.* Internal weakness or injury, on the other hand, tends to produce conditions of deficiency; a deficiency of either *yin* or *yang* produces an excess of the other.

As will be discussed in detail in chapter 8, traditional Chinese medicine classifies diseases according to "symptom-complexes." Two of the major variables that define these symptom-complexes are heat and cold. The relationship of *yin* and *yang* determines which symptom-complex will appear. Usually, a preponderance of *yang* leads to conditions that may be classified as a heat symptom-complex. An overabundance of *yin,* on the other hand, leads to a cold symptom-complex.

Conditions of cold and heat may be either endogenous or exogenous, and they may also produce symptoms on the surface (exterior) or in the depths (interior) of the body. Again, the balance between *yin* and *yang* determines the condition. Thus:

> A deficiency of *yang* brings on exterior cold, while a deficiency of *yin* leads to interior heat. A preponderance of *yang* leads to exterior heat, while a preponderance of *yin* leads to interior cold.
>
> "Treatise on the Regulation of Channels"
> in *Plain Questions*

A deficiency of *yang* resulting in exterior cold means that there is a general hypofunctioning with insufficient body heat. An example is chronic nephritis with symptoms of intolerance to cold, cold limbs, and edema. In this case, the vital function of the spleen and kidney is too weak to perform the functions of transporting and transforming nutrients as well as the proper absorption and elimination of fluids. The result is an accumulation of fluids, dampness, and cold, suggesting deficiency of *yang* and preponderance of *yin*.

A deficiency of *yin* leading to interior heat means that the vital essence is impaired. This impairment produces a relative profusion of *yang* and a state of hyperfunctioning "of a deficient nature." The resulting condition typically includes such symptoms as low fever; a feverish sensation in the palms, the soles, and the region of the chest; flushed cheeks, and night sweats.

A preponderance of *yang* leading to heat manifestation is also a condition of hyperfunctioning, this time with an increase in the body's resistance. This increase in resistance produces surplus heat or leads to an inability to diffuse heat. Such conditions are typical of acute infectious diseases; they are accompanied by a flushed face and temperature above 38° C. The whole body feels hot. Because the excess functioning *(yang)* impairs the body fluid *(yin)*, infectious diseases are also accompanied by thirst, a scant amount of urine, and dry stools. Note that heat conditions can result from either deficiency of *yin* or a preponderance of *yang;* however, they differ in their cause, course, or development and manifestation.

Finally, a preponderance of *yin* leading to interior cold is a functional disturbance or inhibition within the body that results in an accumulation of fluids, dampness, and cold within the body, together with insufficient body heat. This symptom-complex most commonly includes abdominal pain, diarrhea, an intolerance of cold, and an affinity for warmth. The accumulation of cold causes the blood vessels to contract, restricting blood flow. Pain thus occurs. These symptoms appear when the excess *yin* suppresses *yang* (preponderant cold disturbs the vital function) so that it is unable to warm and nourish the muscles. The impairment of *yang* also leads to damage in both the kidney and spleen *yang;* the result is a failure to transport and transform nutrients, which, in turn, leads to diarrhea.

If either *yin* or *yang* becomes extremely impaired, both will become impaired. This pattern in the development of disease follows from the idea that "no *yin* can be formed without *yang*" and that *"yang* fails to come into being without *yin."* Chronic nephritis is a clinical example of this process. The usual symptom of chronic nephritis is edema due to a deficiency of *yang,* which impedes water metabolism. However, at an advanced stage of nephritis, a deficiency of *yin* may also be present if *yang* is too deficient to produce vital substance. The reverse situation occurs in hypertension, which usually begins as a deficiency of *yin* and preponderance of *yang.* As the conditions worsen, however, a deficiency of both *yin* and *yang* may appear. In general, a deficiency of both *yin* and *yang* is most common in cases of chronic disease.

The Intertransformation of Yin and Yang in the Course of Disease

As already indicated, the relationship between *yin* and *yang* changes as a disease progresses. In chronic cases, a deficiency of either *yin* or *yang* usually becomes a deficiency of both. In acute cases, the course of disease is governed by the principle that "extreme *yang* turns into *yin* and extreme *yin* turns into *yang."* That is, the relationship between *yin* and *yang* becomes reversed at some point.

For example, a *yang* symptom-complex of hyperfunction may turn into a *yin* symptom-complex of functional failure. This pattern occurs in patients with pneumonia. They will have symptoms of high fever, flushed face, restlessness, a rapid and forceful pulse, and a marked hyperfunctioning of the body. Such a condition would be readily diagnosed as a symptom-complex of *yang,* excess, and heat, and it would be treated with drugs of a cold nature.

However, if the condition is treated incorrectly or if it is not treated in time, shock due to poisoning may appear. This stage of the disease will be accompanied by sweating, cold limbs, a decrease in body temperature and blood pressure, shortness of breath, a pallid appearance, and a weak and "thready" pulse. This reduction in body response as well as the functional decline represents a symptom-complex of *yin,* deficiency, and cold. Thus extreme *yang* has turned into extreme *yin.*

The appearance of pulmonary infection in patients with chronic asthma is an example of the reverse process—the transformation of *yin* into *yang.* Patients with chronic asthma typically have no fever; the cough produces a whitish, frothy sputum. If such patients are exposed to cold, these symptoms worsen. This condition represents a symptom-complex of *yin* and cold. If a pulmonary infection appears, however, the symptoms will change. Patients will have a fever or aggravated cough with thick, puslike, yellowish sputum, a reddened tongue, and a rapid pulse. Such symptoms indicate that the symptom-complex of *yin* and cold has been transformed into one of *yang* and heat.

Just as conditions of excess and deficiency may be transformed according to the principle of intertransformation of *yin* and *yang,* so the course of disease from the exterior to the interior of the body can be predicted by this principle. For example, the early stages of encephalitis, with fever and an aversion to cold, represent an exterior symptom-complex; if treatment is delayed, the disease will produce high fever, delirium, and convulsions, indicating a transformation to an interior symptom-complex. The reverse may also occur; an interior symptom-complex may transform into an exterior one.

It should be noted that these transformations of excess and deficiency, heat and cold, and exterior and interior conditions depend on a variety of factors. Chief among these are the strength of the body's resistance, the nature of the various pathogenic factors, and the appropriateness and timeliness of treatment. The course of the disease cannot be predicted without taking into account these factors.

Yin and Yang as the Foundation for Diagnosis

A good practitioner differentiates between *yin* and *yang* when observing the complexion and feeling the pulse.

"Treatise on the Correspondence between Man
and the Universe" in *Plain Questions*

In traditional Chinese medicine, there are four diagnostic procedures: looking, listening and smelling, asking, and feeling (including pulse taking). In all of these methods, the first task of the practitioner is to distinguish between *yin* and *yang*.

For example, in looking at the skin, the practitioner should distinguish between a *yang* complexion, which is smooth and glistening, and a *yin* complexion, which is pale or ashen in color. A yellow or red complexion suggests a symptom-complex of *yang* and heat, while a blue and purple, white, or dark color implies a symptom-complex of *yin* and cold.

In listening to a patient, a traditional Chinese practitioner will note whether the voice is sonorous with heavy breathing, which implies a *yang* condition, or whether it is feeble with weak breathing, which suggests a *yin* condition.

Differentiating between *yin* and *yang* is also the essential task of palpating the pulse. Pulses that are floating, overflowing, slippery, or rapid are considered *yang* pulses. Those that are deep, thready, choppy, or slow are *yin* pulses.

The fundamental method for determining the cause, location, and nature of a disease in Chinese medicine is the differentiation of symptom-complexes. While this differentiation is based on several distinctions—namely, the distinctions between heat and cold, exterior and interior, deficiency and excess—the essential distinction is between *yin* and *yang*. All of the others only serve to inform this basic distinction:

—Exterior symptom-complexes of heat and excess are *yang* conditions.
—Interior symptom-complexes of cold and deficiency are *yin* conditions.

Because everything in nature can be described as either *yin* or *yang*—including symptoms of disease—traditional Chinese medicine repeatedly returns to this fundamental distinction in order to determine the nature of the illness. Thus, although clinical pathological conditions may differ in thousands of ways, the differences never exceed the bounds of *yin* and *yang*.

Treatment: Restoring the Balance

Observe the relationship between *yin* and *yang* carefully, and make adjustments to bring about equilibrium.

"General Treatise on the Essential
Principles" in *Plain Questions*

Treat the *yin* aspect for a disease of *yang* nature. Treat the *yang* aspect for a disease of *yin* nature.

"Treatise on the Correspondence Between Man
and the Universe" in *Plain Questions*

In Chinese medicine, the root cause of the occurrence and development of disease is the preponderance or deficiency or *yin* and *yang*. Therefore, the basic principle of therapy is to adjust *yin* and *yang*—to reduce the superfluous, make up the insufficiency, and thereby create conditions that will restore the balance of *yin* and *yang*.

Applying this general principle of restoring balance to the various symptom-complexes, the ancient Chinese arrived at the following guidelines for treatment:

—A cold symptom complex should be treated with drugs that are warm or hot in nature.

—A heat symptom complex should be treated with drugs that are cool or cold in nature.

—A deficiency symptom complex should be treated with a reinforcing method.

—An excess symptom complex should be treated with a reducing method.

Since the use of drugs in Chinese medicine is guided by this principle of restoring the balance of *yin* and *yang,* traditional drugs are also systematically classified according to *yin* and *yang*. Three characteristics of drugs guide this classification: their "basic nature," their flavor, and their effect.

The "basic nature" of a drug may be one of four types: hot, cold, warm, and cool. The *yang* drugs are warm or hot in nature; the *yin* drugs are cool or cold.

There are six classes of flavors. Drugs that are pungent, sweet, and insipid are *yang* drugs; those that are sour, bitter, or salty are *yin* drugs.

Effects fall into one of two primary categories: they are either ascending effects or they are descending effects. Drugs whose effects
are descending, astringent, and, condensing are *yin* drugs. Those
with ascending, floating, and dispersing effects are *yang.*

All of these drugs are administered according to their *yin* or *yang*
nature and the relationship between them and the *yin-yang* nature of
the symptom-complex. The goal, in all cases, is "to reduce what is
superfluous and replenish what is insufficient" to restore the relative
balance of *yin* and *yang* on a new basis.

THE FIVE ELEMENTS: A STUDY OF MOTION

Nothing on earth or within the universe is unrelated to the five elements,
and man is no exception.

"Treatise on the Analysis of *Yin-Yang*
in Twenty-five Different Individuals"
in *Miraculous Pivot*

The second theoretical foundation of traditional Chinese medicine
is the theory of the five elements. This is a theory of systems. It is a
way of describing the internal structure of a system. More important,
however, it is a way of describing the process of change within a
system and between the system and its environment.

In its most basic form, the theory of the five elements is this: All
systems—objects or phenomena—have structural qualities that interact with each other. This interaction produces a constant state of
internal motion, the pattern of which is predictable. All systems in
the universe have the same structural qualities and follow the same
pattern of motion. Hence, it is possible to use analogy to understand
any system; that is, it is possible to use the obvious qualities of one
system to describe the less obvious or hidden qualities of another.

In the theory of the five elements, the ancient Chinese used the
five basic materials familiar in everyday life to symbolize the behavior
of all objects and phenomena in nature. These five elements are:
wood, fire, earth, metal, and water. Each of these elements symbolizes a particular pattern of motion. By analogy to one of these elements, the characteristic movement of any object or phenomenon can
be identified.

The theory of the five elements further describes the relationships
among these five basic patterns of motion—the way one promotes

another or controls it.[2] It also describes the way all five interact in any system to maintain constant motion and growth, as well as the ways in which the relationships may become imbalanced to produce an abnormal pattern of change. The theory of the five elements is thus, above all, a study of motion.

The Motion of the Five Elements

The five elements are water, fire, wood, metal, and earth. Water moistens and flows downward. Fire flares upward. Wood is flexible. Metal may be transformed through casting. And earth serves for the sowing and growing of crops.

"General Regulations" in *The Book of History*

The early Chinese philosophers summarized nature in terms of the five elements. Wood, they said, can be characterized by the process of germination and by a pattern of spreading out freely. Fire symbolizes heat and a pattern of flaring upward. Earth represents the promotion of growth and the process of nourishment. Metal is characterized by purification and solidity. Water is cold and flows downward.

These attributes can be seen in other objects and phenomena in nature. For example, in spring, windy weather prevails. Temperatures increase. It is a time of expansive movement. Trees and grass germinate, giving rise to verdant scenery. Also at this time, fruit is still green and sour. For these reasons, spring, wind, green, sour, and the process of germination are all classified as analogous to wood.

The analogy may be extended to the human body in a similar manner. The human liver, for example, prefers a moist environment. Liver *qi,* it is said, likes to ascend. When diseased, the liver produces symptoms of wind, such as tremors and convulsions. In traditional Chinese medicine, then, the liver is seen as analogous to wood. Its pattern of movement is one of germination and expansion.

In this way, each of the five elements may be used to characterize phenomena in nature. Table 2.1 shows the classification of some of the most common of these phenomena.

2. It should be noted that these relationships apply to the movement of the objects or phenomena, not to their substance. Huang Yuanyu writes in the *Essentials of the four Classics* that "when speaking of the relationship of interpromoting and intercontrolling of the five elements, reference is always made to their *qi* rather than their substances. With regard to substance, it is impossible to talk about promoting or controlling.

TABLE 2.1. Classification of Phenomena in Nature According to the Theory of the Five Elements

Five Elements	Phenomena in Nature					Phenomena in Human Body				
	Five Colors	Climatic Factors	Growth and Development	Seasons	Five Flavors	Zang Organ	Fu Organ	Sense Organs	Tissues	Emotion
Wood	Green	Wind	Germination	Spring	Sour	Liver	Gallbladder	Eye	Tendon	Anger
Fire	Red	Heat	Growth	Summer	Bitter	Heart	Small intestine	Tongue	Vessel	Joy
Earth	Yellow	Dampness	Transformation	Late summer	Sweet	Spleen	Stomach	Mouth	Muscle	Pensiveness
Metal	White	Dryness	Reaping	Autumn	Pungent	Lung	Large intestine	Nose	Skin and hair	Grief
Water	Black	Cold	Storing	Winter	Salty	Kidney	Urinary bladder	Ear	Bone	Fear

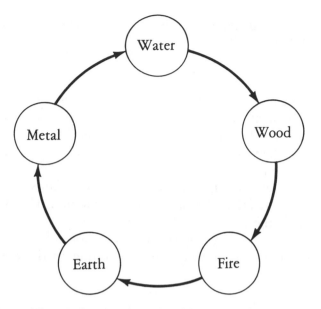

FIGURE 2.1.   The Mother-Son Relationship among the Five Elements

The Mother-Son Relationship

Each of the five elements has its own characteristic motion. But none acts alone. Rather, all systems contain all five elements, and all five are interrelated. The theory recognizes two basic types of relationship: promoting relationships and controlling relationships. The promoting relationship is known as the "mother-son" relationship.

The mother element promotes—or gives birth to—the son element. The son cannot promote the mother directly. Thus, the mother-son relationship defines a cycle of change that occurs in a specific direction and order: wood promotes fire; fire promotes earth; earth promotes metal; metal promotes water; water, in turn, promotes wood. This cycle is shown in figure 2.1.

Relationships of Control

With metal, wood is felled. With water, fire is extinguished. With wood, earth is rooted and loosened. With fire, metal is melted. And with earth,

water is obstructed. This is the relationship among objects, too numerous
to mention individually.

"Treatise on How to Keep Healthy"
in *Plain Questions*

The second major relationship is one of control. In this relationship, each element occupies both a position of "actor" and one of
"being acted on." Like the mother-son relationship, control proceeds
in a defined order: wood acts on earth; earth acts on water; water
acts on fire; fire acts on metal; and metal acts on wood.

When both relationships are operating in a system simultaneously,
they produce a relatively stable internal structure. This structure is
represented by the diagram in figure 2.2.

These two relationships—promotion and control—are inseparable
traits of all objects and phenomena, according to the theory of the

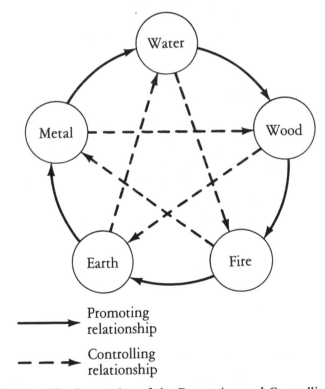

FIGURE 2.2.   The Interaction of the Promoting and Controlling Relationships among the Five Elements

five elements. Without promotion, there would be no birth and development. Without control, equilibrium and harmony in the development and change of things could not be maintained. Thus, neither is dispensable. The two relationships, like *yin* and *yang,* are mutually supporting and restraining.

Because no element in this system is isolated from another, a change in one is bound to influence another (and to be influenced by another). Therefore, the condition of any one of the parts reflects the condition of all of the other parts. Since each element is also always in motion, all of the elements are in motion. Viewed as a whole, however, the system appears to be in a state of equilibrium. This is the dynamic balance that traditional Chinese thought describes as the condition necessary for the normal growth and development of things:

> In the mystery of nature, neither promotion of growth nor control is dispensable. Without promotion of growth, there would be no development; without control, excessive growth would result in harm.
>
> *Illustrated Supplement to the Classic*
> *of Categories*

Feedback: Maintaining a Healthy Imbalance

> Where control *qi* appears, reaction *qi* also appears; then control *qi* comes again. Without reaction *qi,* harm would result.
>
> "General Treatise on the Essential Principles"
> in *Plain Questions*

The mother-son relationship creates a cycle of effects in which one element promotes another. The control relationship creates another, different cycle in which one element controls another. If these cycles are viewed individually, it appears that the relationship between any two elements is always unidirectional. Wood always promotes fire, but fire never promotes wood. Earth controls water, but water cannot control earth.

However, in reality, the two cycles operate simultaneously, and their simultaneous operation creates a feedback mechanism. Through this feedback mechanism, the relationship between any two elements becomes reciprocal.

The feedback mechanism works in the following way: Fire is controlled by water, but it cannot directly control water. It can, however, promote the growth of earth, and earth can control water. Thus, by promoting the growth of earth, fire creates a *controlling reaction* on water so that water does not overly restrain fire and fire does not decline.

At the same time, fire is both promoted by wood and promotes the growth of earth; the latter action strengthens the restraint of earth upon water, weakening the promotion of wood by water, thus reducing the potential overpromotion of fire by wood. In this way, fire is controlled.

In a system, then, an element can only promote another element if it also indirectly controls it. These indirect relationships are as follows:

—Wood promotes the growth of fire by controlling earth.[3]
—Fire promotes the growth of earth by controlling metal.
—Earth promotes the growth of metal by controlling water.
—Metal promotes the growth of water by controlling wood.
—Water promotes the growth of wood by controlling fire.

This feedback system establishes a continuous process of consuming and gaining, during which an imbalance between these two—that is, between consuming and gaining—often appears. The imbalance is an adjustment. These adjustments follow a cycle in which balance is obtained within an imbalance and then immediately replaced by a new imbalance.

The feedback system can itself become imbalanced if there is too large an imbalance between two elements—that is, if the normal promoting and controlling relationships are disturbed in some way. There is, however, a mechanism for restoring imbalance in this situation. It is known as the control-reaction mechanism.

This mechanism is the result of the cyclic interplay of two forces: control *qi* and reaction *qi*. Control *qi* is the excessive control of one element over another and appears when either the promoting rela-

---

3. In the cycle of promoting and controlling relationships, earth can promote the growth of metal only when controlled by wood. Metal in turn controls wood, guaranteeing the normal functioning of the latter and promoting the growth of fire. Chinese medicine holds that excessive activity of the five elements will inevitably impede the normal promotion of growth.

tionship is insufficient or the controlling relationship is excessive. This control *qi,* in turn, induces the appearance of its opposite— reaction *qi.*

For example, when fire as a controlling factor is excessive and overrestrains metal, the latter becomes too weak to control wood. Wood becomes preponderant and increases its restraint over earth, so that earth will not check water. Water will then become exuberant and bring fire back to normal. This cycle is illustrated in figure 2.3.

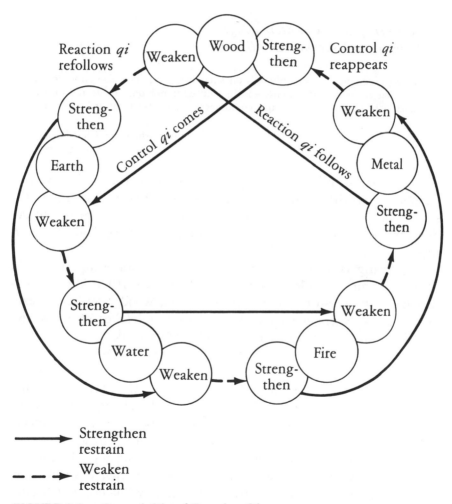

FIGURE 2.3. Control *Qi* and Reaction *Qi*

Notice that this sequence of effects is different from that of the normal feedback mechanism. There thus exist two mechanisms for spontaneous adjustment in a system. Under normal conditions the relationships of promoting and controlling, working in harmony, adjust the motion of the system. Under abnormal conditions, when the promoting and controlling relationships are severely disrupted, these relationships themselves are adjusted by the control-reaction mechanism.

Overacting and Counteracting: Response to External Conditions

> Being excessive, *qi* not only acts on what it should, but also counteracts on what it should not. Being insufficient, *qi* is not only overacted on by what acts upon it, but is also counteracted upon by what it should act on.
>
> "Treatise on the Five Circuit Phases"
> in *Plain Questions*

The dynamic balance of a system may be disturbed by external factors. When this occurs, the relationships between elements in the system become destructive. The theory of the five elements recognizes two kinds of destructive relationships: *overacting* and *counteracting*.

Overacting is a type of excessive control. It can occur in cases of deficiency; for example, wood will overact on earth if the latter is deficient. Or it can occur in cases of excess; wood may be too exuberant to be restrained by metal and thus unleashes an aggressive invasion against earth, which in turn becomes weak.

Counteracting reverses the normal controlling relationship between pairs of elements. It, too, can arise from either deficiency or excess. For example, an element may be exuberant beyond restraint; its movement counteracts the movement of the element that should be controlling it. For example, wood should be controlled by metal; but if it is too exuberant to be restrained, it will instead counteract metal and begin to control it. In the case of deficiency, the element is so weak that it is counteracted by the element that it should control. Wood should control earth, but if it is weakened by external influences, earth will instead begin to control wood. These relation-

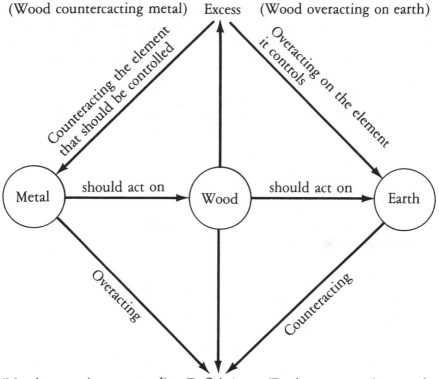

(Wood countercacting metal)   Excess   (Wood overacting on earth)

(Metal overacting on wood)   Deficiency   (Earth counteracting wood)

FIGURE 2.4.   **Overacting and Counteracting Relationships among the Five Elements**

ships, which are illustrated in figure 2.4, represent an imbalance that cannot be spontaneously adjusted by the system. In the human body, they represent disease.

THE FIVE ELEMENTS AND THE HUMAN BODY

The theory of the five elements is a general statement about the structure and functioning of objects in nature. The human body is no exception to this generalization. In traditional Chinese medicine, the five-element theory is used to explain the physiology of the body as well as its relationship to the environment.

The human body is a system. It is composed of structural elements—organs and tissues—that are analogous to the five elements. The interaction of these organs and tissues proceeds according to the pattern of relationships among the five elements. As a system, the body is also related to environmental conditions, such as the seasons and climatic factors; the theory of the five elements helps to explain these relationships as well. It outlines the basic pattern of the transmission of disease, sets forth guidelines for diagnosis, and defines an approach to treatment that takes into account the interaction of all the elements of the system.

The Zang Organs: The Five Fundamental Elements of the Body

As will be described in the next chapter, traditional Chinese medicine views the five *zang* organs as the center of physiological activity of the human body. These five organs are analogous to the five elements. And like the five elements, the *zang* organs are all interrelated in relationships of promotion and control.

For example, the liver corresponds to wood. It is thus promoted by the kidney (water) while it promotes the heart (fire). It is controlled by the lung (metal) and, in turn, controls the spleen (earth).

These interrelationships help to explain the functions of the internal organs and their interrelationships. While these functional relationships will be discussed in detail in chapter 3, they can be summarized as follows:

—The kidney (water) stores essence and nourishes the liver.
—The liver (wood) stores blood and supplies the heart.
—The heart (fire) produces heat and warms the spleen.
—The spleen (earth) transforms and conveys the essence of food to replenish the lung
—The lung (metal) aids in providing the kidney with water through its descending movement.

These relationships among the *zang* organs correspond to the promoting relationships among the five elements. The organs also function in controlling relationships:

—The upward-moving overexuberant liver *yang* can be inhibited by the descending lung *qi* (metal controls wood).

—Stagnation of the spleen in transporting can be overcome by the smooth flow of liver *qi* (wood controls earth).

—Edema due to deficiency of the kidney *yang* can be checked by the normal transporting and transforming function of the spleen (earth controls water).

—A flaring up of the heart fire can be prevented by the moistening action of the kidney (water controls fire).

—Excessive descending movement of the lung can be controlled by the heat of the heart (fire controls metal).

Overacting and Counteracting: The Transmission of Disease

Overacting and counteracting are the destructive relationships that emerge when external factors disrupt the normal balance of a system. In the body, these destructive relationships, together with the basic mother-son relationship, explain the way in which disease is transmitted among the internal organs.

Figure 2.5 illustrates the transmission of disease to and from the liver. The liver is the mother in the mother-son relationship with the heart. Excessive liver *yang* may thus induce exuberant fire in the heart marked by dizziness, giddiness, a reddened tongue, insomnia, and irritability. The transmission of liver trouble to the heart is thus known as "a disorder of the mother element affecting the son element."

The liver normally controls the spleen. A dysfunction in the travel of *qi* due to a stagnant liver will produce excessive control or "over-acting" on the spleen, so that it is unable to convey nutrients and water through the body. This condition, known as "wood overacting on earth," produces symptoms such as lack of appetite, abdominal distension, and diarrhea.

The liver can also transmit disease to its mother element, the kidney. In this case the upward exuberance of liver *yang* that produces a hyperactivity of fire leads to overconsumption of kidney *yin* (water). The typical symptoms are dizziness and spermatorrhea.

Finally, the liver is normally controlled by the lung. However, the so-called "flaring up" of liver fire may create a counteracting relationship with the lung. The result is pulmonary disease with

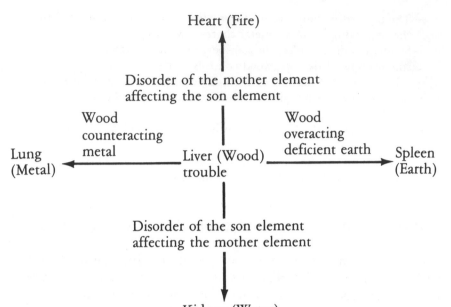

FIGURE 2.5.   Transmission of Disease to and from the Liver

symptoms of cough, pain in the chest, and coughing up of blood.

These patterns of transmission of disease—overacting, counteracting, and pathological transmission between mother and son elements—do not *necessarily* occur. The development of destructive relationships depends on the condition of the individual. Weak organs may be affected, but strong ones may not. Thus, the theory does not absolutely predict the path of disease, but rather suggests the possible paths it might take.

The Five Elements as a Guide to Diagnosis and Treatment

Knowledge through visual inspection means that the nature of a disease can be discovered by observing the "five colors" of the patient. Knowledge through listening indicates that diseases can be distinguished by listening to the "five tones" of the patient. Knowledge through inquiry refers to the practice of asking about the "five tastes" that the patient prefers, to determine the cause and location of the disease. Knowledge through pulse-taking differentiates the conditions of deficiency and excessiveness, and determines in which organ the disease is located.

"The Sixty-First Problem" in *Classic on Medical
Problems*

Traditional Chinese medicine identifies the abnormal functioning of the internal organs by noting, in particular, the patient's complexion, quality of voice, taste preferences, and pulse conditions. Traditional practitioners use the theory of the five elements to interpret observations systematically.

For example, the analogies presented earlier in table 2.1 suggest that a green tinge in the complexion, accompanied by pain and distension in the upper gastric region, a preference for sour food, and a taut pulse, indicates liver trouble. Or a florid complexion, accompanied by a bitter taste in the mouth, ulcers or reddening on the tip of the tongue, and overflowing or rapid pulse, suggest an overabundance of heart fire.

These signs can also be interpreted by applying an understanding of the relationships among the five elements. Thus a recognized deficiency in the spleen, accompanied by a livid face and sour regurgitation, indicates that the liver (wood) is overacting on the spleen (earth).

Such diagnoses, which reflect an understanding of the pattern of transmission of disease from one organ to another, have important implications for the treatment of the condition.

In fact, it is a characteristic of traditional Chinese medicine to treat not only the diseased organ itself, but also the related organ. For instance, the five-element theory suggests that liver trouble may well spread to the spleen; the therapeutic strategy is thus to tonify the spleen to prevent transmission. Or the practitioner may directly treat one organ in order to influence the condition of the diseased organ. For example, the five-element theory outlines the following treatment methods:

- Replenish water (kidney) to supply wood (liver)
- Increase earth (spleen) to promote metal (lung)
- Sustain earth (spleen) to check wood (liver)
- Strengthen water (kidney) to inhibit fire (heart)

Finally, the five-element theory also guides the use of medicinal herbs. The colors and flavors of drugs can correspond to the five *zang* organs (though they do not always). For example, red drugs might be expected to act on the heart. Sour drugs are said to act on the liver.

The theory of the five elements, then, has played a major historical role in understanding clinical experience and in the development of the theory of traditional Chinese medicine. As a theory, it compels the practitioner to observe the human body as a structured system and therefore to try to understand the organic connection between the different parts of the body as well as unity between the body and the environmental conditions in which it exists. With its emphasis on dynamic balance, it has led to a medical theory that sees disease as a breakdown in the equilibrium among internal parts of the body and between the body and environment. The essential task of the Chinese practitioner is to seek the cause and mechanism of the imbalance in a patient and then to seek the therapy and medication that will restore the balance. The theory of *yin* and *yang* provides the basic principle of treatment for Chinese medicine: namely, to attain an integrated balance of the body by adjusting the relationship of *yin* and *yang*. The theory of the five elements, though, specifies the types of adjustments that are possible and necessary.

RECOGNIZING LIMITS AND SETTING NEW DIRECTIONS

While modern theorists of traditional Chinese medicine recognize its clinical effectiveness, they are also aware that the theories of *yin-yang* and the five elements are, to some extent, limited in their ability to contribute to a scientific understanding of medical phenomena. Contemporary Chinese theorists identify two limitations in particular. The first is a problem of the level of generalization. The second is a lack of understanding of what is called "upward spiraling."

Regarding the question of level of generalization, for example, modern writers point out that the type of opposition implied in the theory of *yin-yang* is only one of the classes of oppositions. In contemporary Chinese thought, any unity of opposition within an object or phenomenon is termed "contradiction." This contradiction places no limits on the nature of either of the opposing aspects. In the theory of *yin-yang,* however, the opposing aspects have fixed and invariable qualities. This assignment of specific characteristics to *yin* and *yang* limits the range of generalization; it cannot be applied as widely as the more general theory of dialectics.

This same limitation also applies to the traditional understanding of the nature of the relationship between opposites. In the theory of *yin* and *yang,* the relationship of interdependence, transformation, and conflict are limited to what can be perceived directly through the senses. A more sophisticated theory would be able to characterize the more abstract qualities of these relationships, such as the relativity of the unity of opposites or the absoluteness of conflict.

The theory of the five elements has similar limitations. It describes a structural pattern that can be universally applied to all systems, based upon a simple, fixed arrangement of a small number of elements with specific properties (namely, those defined by wood, fire, earth, metal, and water). But as in the case of *yin-yang,* the assignment of these fixed properties limits the ability to explain the relationships among objects and phenomena in nature. Such a theory can potentially restrain the thinking of those who would summarize more general principles based on new findings. The theory of the five elements cannot, therefore, be viewed as the complete general theory of systems.

Both the theory of *yin-yang* and the theory of the five elements explain change over time. Both characterize this change as cyclic in nature. Yet neither explains the process of *spiraling upward.* Clearly, some types of change involve the development from a lower to a higher level. Contemporary Chinese theorists see a need to integrate a description of this law of upward spiraling with the more traditional descriptions of periodic cycles in the theories of *yin* and *yang* and the five elements.

Modern researchers of traditional Chinese medicine note that it is particularly important to study the theories of *yin* and *yang* and the five elements with the help of modern scientific technology, including modern medicine and some related sciences such as cybernetics and systems theory. Such study would focus on the material basis for the theories of *yin-yang* and the five elements in human physiology and pathology. For example, recent developments in the study of the endocrine system have provided good ground for study on the theories of *yin-yang* and the five elements, and are therefore worth studying in a comparative manner. Also, the connections between systems within the human body deserve special attention.

IN SUMMARY

The theories of *yin* and *yang* and the five elements form the philosophical foundation of traditional Chinese medicine. Both of these theories are theories of change and development. The theory of *yin* and *yang* describes the process by which phenomena with opposing qualities interact to form an integrated whole. The theory of the five elements provides a framework for viewing the elements of any system, the relationship between these elements, and the pattern of motion that results from their interaction.

Applied to the human body, the theory of *yin* and *yang* provides a model for the development of disease. In a healthy body, *yin* and *yang* are continuously consuming and supporting each other; they produce a dynamic equilibrium in the body. If this balance is disrupted, however, an excess or deficiency of either *yin* or *yang* leads to a state of illness.

The theory of the five elements provides a model for the interaction among the organs of the body and for the transmission of disease when one of them fails to function properly. Each of the *zang* and *fu* organs corresponds to one of the five elements. The relationship among the five elements is thus a picture of the relationship among the organs. It is also the path that disease is most likely to follow.

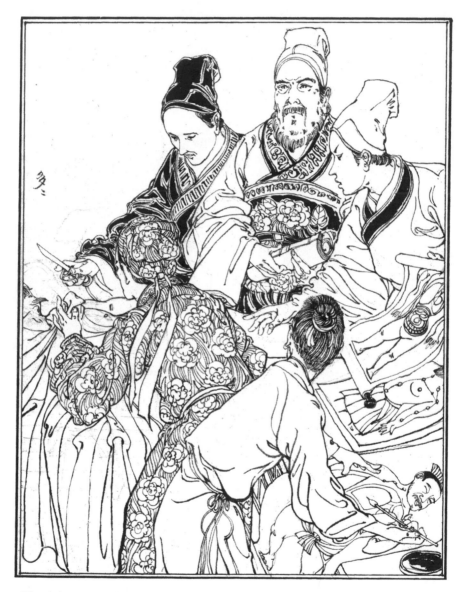

Physicians examining anatomical organs during surgery.

———————————◆·◆———————————

CHAPTER THREE

The *Zang-Fu* System

Zang is seated in the interior, yet it manifests on the exterior. Hence, it is called the "organ picture." [1]

Classic of Categories

THE THEORY OF the *zang-fu* system is at the core of traditional Chinese medicine. *Zang* means "organ." However, while the heart, liver, spleen, lung, and kidney share the same names in both Chinese and Western medicine, the concept of an organ in Chinese medicine is not the same as in Western science.

For the Chinese, each organ is a system that might best be described as an energy network. This network includes the structures that Western medicine calls organs. But it also includes other tissues such as skin, muscle, tendons, and bones as well as the sense organs—the eyes, ears, mouth, and nose. In addition, the concept of organ includes the pathways which interconnect these various parts of the body. These form the channel system. When Chinese medicine speaks of the heart, for example, it is speaking of this whole system and the functions it performs.

This meaning of "organ" leads to four important concepts. The first is the definition of life. According to traditional Chinese medi-

---

1. "Organ picture" does not refer to a diagram of the internal organs. Instead, "organ picture" expresses the idea that the functions of the internal organs can be observed on the exterior of the body. By using the term "organ picture," Chineses medical theorists assert that it is possible to deduce the physiological and pathological changes of the interior of the body from outward signs.

cine, *life is a reflection of the activity of the organs, including their associated channels.* Each organ has its own attributes and functions. Together their activity produces the four basic life materials: essence, *qi,* blood, and body fluid. These materials, in turn, make possible the activity of the individual organs.

The second concept is that of "relationship." The theory of the *zang-fu* organs does not explain the body solely in terms of the characteristics and functions of the various organs. Just as important are the relationships between the *zang* and *fu* organs and among the five *zang* organs, as well as the relationships between the exterior and interior portions of the body and the upper and lower halves of the body. These relationships conform to the principles of the theories of *yin* and *yang* and of the five elements.

Third is the concept of "multiple functions." In Chinese medicine, one organ may perform many functions. For example, the heart not only "governs blood circulation and the vessels," but also "stores consciousness." It thus carries out some of the functions of the nervous system in Western medicine, especially that of the cerebral cortex.

Finally, the traditional Chinese definition of disease is an imbalance in the *zang-fu* system. Since the *zang-fu* organs form a network over the entire body, they oppose each other and unify each other into a whole at the same time. They are interdependent; each depends on the other for its functioning. They also restrain each other, blocking each other's functions. A relative balance and harmony between the organs must exist if these relationships are to be maintained. Disease occurs when the balance is disrupted. Such a disruption may result from factors in both the internal and external environment.

The theory of the *zang-fu* system is thus the theory of (1) the basic life materials; (2) the way these materials are used and produced by the organs of the body; (3) the relationships that keep the system operating; and (4) the disease that occurs when the relationships fail.

THE BASIC LIFE MATERIALS

The four basic substances of life are essence, *qi,* blood, and body fluid.

Essence

> Essence is essential for the construction of the body.
>
> "Treatise on the Essential Laws of Disease
> Occurrence" in *Plain Questions*

Essence is the fundamental material—the source—of living organisms. It is of two types: congenital (or innate) essence, and acquired essence. Congenital essence is received from one's parents; it is also known as reproductive essence or "essence that exists before birth." Acquired essence develops from food, air, and water following birth. The two types are interdependent and promote each other. Congential essence provides the fundamental materials for the later development of acquired essence, and is present before birth; after birth, acquired essence continues to nourish congenital essence, replenishing and invigorating it. Essence can be transformed into *qi*—that is, into energy or movement—thus helping to maintain life activity.

Qi

> Man relies on *qi* and nutrients to stay alive.
>
> "Treatise on How to Keep Healthy"
> in *Plain Questions*

Qi has many faces in traditional Chinese medicine. The predominant one is a rarefied substance that is constantly in motion. The movement of *qi* is literally the activity of life. At the same time, because it is a substance, *qi* is also viewed as one of the fundamental materials for the construction of the body.

The *qi* that circulates throughout the body is the most vigorous form of *qi*. It has four basic patterns of movement: ascending, descending, exiting, and entering. The channels are the passageways along which these movements occur.

In addition to activating the body, *qi* performs several other functions. It warms the body and defends it against pathogenic factors. It also constrains the blood and body fluid to their proper vessels. Finally, it transforms the other basic life materials. As it performs these functions, it changes character. For example, *yang qi* is the form of *qi* that warms the body. It regulates body temperature. A deficiency of *yang qi* results in symptoms such as chills and cold limbs.

Finally, *qi* is also the actual activity—the physiological functioning—of the organs, channels, and tissues. Thus, liver *qi,* for instance, is the action of the liver in the body.

Other forms of *qi* are defined by their distribution, their origin, and their specific functions. For example:

—Original *qi* is also known as genuine *qi.* It derives from a combination of congenital essence and acquired essence derived from food, water, and air. Original *qi* exists everywhere; it surrounds the organs and tissues of the body's interior and is found in the interstitial spaces between the skin and muscles on the exterior of the body. It is disseminated through the body by the Triple Burner.

—*Wei qi* defends the surface layer of the body to guard against any invasion by external pathogenic factors. It is transformed from food essence and is actually a part of *yang qi,* sometimes called "defensive *yang.*" Its circulation is not controlled by the vessels; rather, it travels through the skin and flesh, scattering systemically. It performs its defensive function by controlling the opening and closing of pores, by helping to regulate body temperature, and by moistening the skin.

—Pectoral *qi* is a combination of the air inhaled and the food essence that has been transformed by the stomach and spleen and stored in the chest. Its main function is to propel respiration and the beating of the heart in order to promote the circulation of blood.

—Nourishing *qi* is rarefied substance produced from food collected and transformed by the spleen and stomach. It flows through the blood vessels and becomes a component of blood, circulating throughout the body and supplying it with nutrients.

Blood

Blood and *qi* are the basis of mentality.
"Treatise on Seasonal Changes and Vitality"
in *Plain Questions*

The third basic life material is blood—the red fluid that circulates in the vessels. As indicated, blood is a product of nourishing *qi,* transformed from food essence. It transports nutrients to the entire body, including the internal organs and the body's flesh and bones, thus allowing them to perform their individual functions.

Blood is also considered by Chinese medicine to be the material basis for mental activities. When a person has an abundance of *qi* and blood, his or her thinking will be clear and vigorous.

Body Fluid

Body fluid is the fourth basic substance of life. In traditional Chinese medicine, it refers to all the fluids in the body, including saliva, stomach fluids, synovial fluids, and tissue fluids. It also refers to such secretions as tears, nasal mucous, sweat, and urine that has not yet been discharged. The most important function of body fluid is to keep the skin, flesh, and internal organs moist. It also moistens the body orifices, lubricates the joints, and nourishes the bone and brain marrows.[2] Furthermore, the proper elimination of wastes, the maintenance of a normal body temperature, and the regulation of the balance of *yin* and *yang* in the body all depend on body fluid.

The process of formation, transmission, dissemination, and elimination of body fluid results from the coordinated activity of the various organs, but especially the lung, spleen, and kidney.

These four substances are closely related. They promote, restrain, and permeate each other; they even transform themselves one into the other. For example, *qi* can produce blood, activating it and governing its circulation. Blood and *qi* circulate together, which leads Chinese medicine to label blood the "mother of *qi*." *Qi* can also be transformed into body fluid. Like blood, body fluid is bound to *qi* and circulates with it. If body fluid is impeded, *qi* is also obstructed and fails to function. The result is a deficiency of blood, which, in turn, reduces essence, since blood and essence have a common source.

Together and separately, essence, *qi*, blood, and body fluid thus support the basic activities of life—the functions of the *zang-fu* organs.

---

2. Brain marrow refers to the spinal marrow that permeates the brain. (See "The Kidney Produces Marrow" in this chapter.)

ZANG AND *FU*: THE INTERNAL / EXTERNAL RELATIONSHIP

Original *qi* is kept in the five *zang* organs without discharge; hence, the *zang* organ is full, but not stagnant.

"Further Discussions on the Five *Zang* Organs"
in *Plain Questions*

The six *fu* organs transform food into essence, but do not store it.

"Further Discussions on the Five *Zang* Organs"
in *Plain Questions*

Chinese medicine recognizes two classes of organs: the *zang* and the *fu*.

There are five *zang* organs: the heart, liver, spleen, lung, and kidney. Their function is to transform and store original *qi*. The basic life processes are constantly consuming this rarefied substance. But the supply of *qi* is also constantly being replenished. The task of the *zang* organs is to maintain a full and vital supply of *qi*. If they fail—if *qi* becomes stagnant—illness occurs.

The second class of organs is the *fu* organs. These include the gallbladder, stomach, small and large intestines, urinary bladder, and Triple Burner. They digest, absorb, and excrete. Their function is to take in and digest food, differentiating the usable from the unusable and then discharging the waste products. Unlike the *zang* organs, the *fu* organs are continuously cleared of their contents. If they are not—if they are full of unusable material—disease develops.[3]

In contrasting the *zang* and *fu* organs, traditional Chinese medicine says the *zang* organs "store without discharging," while the *fu*

---

3. This pattern of discharge without storage was noted in the *Classic of Internal Medicine*, which states: "After taking in food, the stomach is full and the intestine empty; as the food moves downward, the intestine becomes full and the stomach empty." Later, Chinese medical theorists came to assert that "it is necessary to keep the *fu* organs clear." More recently, this idea has led clinical researchers to study the effectiveness of purgation for treating such acute abdominal diseases as appendicitis, intestinal obstruction, and gallstones. Preliminary experimental results suggest that herbal remedies such as the Drastic Purgative Decoction act directly on the muscles of the intestinal wall to promote peristalsis and relieve intussusception. Another prescription known as the Decoction for Expelling Stones from the Bile Duct flushes stones from the biliary duct by relaxing the choledochal sphincter and increasing bile secretion.

TABLE 3.1. Summary of the *Zang-fu* System

Five Zang Organs	Five Fu Organs	Five Tissues	Sense Organs and Orifices	Channels	Storage of	Related Emotion
Heart	Small intestine	Vessel	Tongue	Heart channel of hand-shaoyin, small intestine channel of hand-taiyang	Consciousness	Joy
Liver	Gallbladder	Tendon	Eye	Liver channel of foot-jueyin, gallbladder channel of foot-shaoyang	Soul	Anger
Spleen	Stomach	Muscle	Mouth	Spleen channel of foot-taiyin, stomach channel of foot-yangming	Intention	Pensiveness
Lung	Large intestine	Skin	Nose	Lung channel of hand-taiyin, large intestine channel of hand-yangming	Vitality	Grief
Kidney	Urinary bladder	Bone	Ear, genitals and anus	Kidney channel of foot-shaoyin, urinary bladder channel of foot-taiyang	Determination	Terror

organs "discharge with storing."[4] The *zang* organs are relatively solid, while the *fu* are hollow. The *zang* are classified as *yin* (because they resemble the solidity of the earth); the *fu* are classified as *yang* (because they resemble the movement of heaven). Finally, the *zang* organs are viewed as interior in terms of their location in the body. In contrast, the *fu* organs are considered relatively exterior organs.

Zang and *fu* are thus opposing but related organs. They work in pairs. Each *zang* organ is bound in a so-called "exterior/interior" relationship with one *fu* organ.[5] If one fails, the other will suffer also. Table 3.1 summarizes these relationships and describes the other tissues and organs that are associated with each pair.

THE FUNCTIONS OF THE *ZANG-FU* ORGANS

The theory of the *zang-fu* organs is a way of describing the activities of the body. Traditional Chinese medicine does not often speak of the size, shape, and composition of the organs or of the mechanisms by which they operate. Rather, it speaks about their functions—what they do and how they are related to other parts of the body. These functions are explained as follows.

The Heart and the Small Intestine

The heart is the master of the *zang-fu* organs.
"Treatise on Exogenous Pathogenic Factors and
Treatment" in *Miraculous Pivot*

The heart is the ruling member of the *zang-fu* organs. It controls the life processes of the human body, coordinating the activities of all the other organs. In addition:

4. This does not imply that the *zang* organs never discharge or that there is never any movement of the substances they store. The substances or essences of the *zang* organs must constantly be replenished and in abundance. Nor does the fact that there is "no storage" in the *fu* organs indicate their inability to keep what they store. The main function of the *fu* organs is discharging instead of storing their contents.

5. Chinese medicine usually speaks of six *fu* organs, but only five *zang* organs. The sixth *fu* organ is the Triple Burner. It interacts with the pericardium—the envelope surrounding the heart—which is sometimes called a *zang* organ. The Triple Burner-pericardium pair differs from the other *zang-fu* organs in that it plays a subsidiary role to the small intestine/heart in the set of relationships defined by the five elements.

THE HEART GOVERNS THE BLOOD AND VESSELS.

The blood vessels are connected to the heart. Blood flows through them under the power of heart *qi.* If a person is full of vigor, the heart is probably functioning well, with the blood circulating smoothly to transport nutrients to all parts of the body. The vitality of heart *qi* can be determined by changes in the pulse, which indicates the frequency and rhythm of the heartbeat. When heart *qi* is abundant and the blood vessels are full, the pulse beats smoothly and forcefully. When heart *qi* is insufficient, the pulse is weak.

THE HEART CONTROLS MENTAL ACTIVITIES.

In Chinese medicine, mental activity is a general term for the life processes. In its broadest sense, it refers to the outward activities of life; in a more narrow sense, it refers to such activities as perception and thinking. In contrast to Western science, which holds that these activities are controlled by the brain and specifically by the cerebral cortex, traditional Chinese medicine says that it is the heart that governs these activities. The brain is seen primarily as an organ that receives and stores impressions:

> The ears, eyes, mouth and nose are seated in the head, the highest part of the body; this location allows things to be taken in easily. Thus, the brain is the first to receive an impression and feel its existence; it then deposits the impression in its memory.
>
> *The Origin of Medicine*

Mental disorders arise when the heart is injured in some way. For example, some infectious diseases will cause delirium and derangement. Chinese medicine explains that this disorder results when pathogenic factors invade the pericardium, which is the outer sac that surrounds and protects the heart.

THE CONDITION OF THE HEART MAY BE SEEN IN THE CONDITION OF THE COMPLEXION.

Because the face has an abundance of blood vessels, the complexion can reveal the condition of the heart (since the heart governs the vessels). When heart *qi* is abundant, the complexion is ruddy and lustrous; when it is insufficient, the face is pale.

THE HEART IS LINKED TO THE TONGUE.

Chinese medicine says that "the tongue is the body opening of the heart." It also says that "a normal tongue can taste because it is supplied by heart *qi*."

THE HEART AND SMALL INTESTINE FORM A *ZANG-FU* PAIR.

The small intestine has the function of "receiving and containing" water and food. It "converts food into useful substances" and "differentiates the usable from the unusable." In other words, the small intestine takes in the food that the stomach has digested in a preliminary way; it digests it further, differentiating the rarefied substances from the unusable. This organ also assimilates nutrients or "food essence," which is eventually transported to various parts of the body. It sends solid wastes to the large intestine and liquid wastes through the kidney to the urinary bladder to be expelled from the body.[6]

The Liver and the Gallbladder

> The liver stores blood, and the heart promotes its circulation. Blood travels along the channels when the human body is active, but during rest, it returns to the liver. Thus, the liver is known as the "reservoir of blood."
>
> "Treatise on the Relationship between
> Outward Manifestations and the *Zang* Organs"
> in *Plain Questions*

The liver performs the following functions:

THE LIVER STORES BLOOD.

By controlling the storage of blood, the liver regulates the volume of blood that is in circulation at any given time. When the body is active, the demand for blood increases. The liver is the organ that allows this demand to be met.

---

6. These functions include many attributed by Western medicine to the circulatory system, the cerebral cortex of the central nervous system, and the autonomic nervous system.

THE LIVER REGULATES THE FLOW OF *QI*.

Traditional Chinese medicine says that the liver "favors a smooth flow of *qi* and has an aversion to stagnancy." This smooth flow of *qi,* in turn, serves two functions. First, it regulates emotional activities; when liver *qi* does not flow smoothly and is obstructed, abnormal emotional activities such as depression or moodiness may result. Second, the smooth flow of *qi* ensures that the digestive processes operate normally. The unimpeded flow of liver *qi* not only helps regulate the spleen and stomach *qi* so that these organs can perform normally; it also controls the secretion of bile. If liver *qi* does not flow smoothly, the spleen and stomach may function irregularly, and the secretion and elimination of bile may become abnormal. As a result, dyspepsia or jaundice can occur. In addition to maintaining normal emotion and digestive activity, the smooth flow of liver *qi* guarantees the orderly functioning of the Triple Burner and the so-called "water passageway."[7] When liver *qi* is impeded due to liver trouble, channels may be obstructed by stagnated blood, and fluid may accumulate, resulting in ascites.

THE LIVER STORES THE SOUL.[8]

In traditional Chinese medicine, the spirit includes the whole of mental activity. Part of this activity is the soul, and this part is stored in the liver. The spirit—or mental activity—permits the body to react to a variety of situations. When the spirit is at ease, the soul is calm. When the spirit is disturbed, so is the soul. A disturbance of the soul leads to excessive dreaming during sleep or to timidity and trance. Since the liver stores the soul, the composure of the soul and of the spirit as a whole are believed to be dependent on the smooth flow of liver *qi*. Depression or stagnation of liver *qi* readily

7. The "water passageway" is the Triple Burner, three portions of the body cavity that may be compared to water communications. The "water passageway" is the foundation and controller of the circulation of body fluids.

8. The liver in traditional Chinese medicine serves a variety of functions that are served by several organs and systems in Western medicine. Specifically, it involves functions attributed by Western medicine to both the central and autonomic nervous system, to the musculoskeletal system, to the circulatory system, and to the organs of vision, as well as to the liver and gallbladder of Western medicine.

causes suspicion and anger. A restless soul, according to traditional Chinese medicine, leads to raving.

THE LIVER CONTROLS THE CONDITION OF THE TENDONS.

The tendons connect muscles with their body attachments and aid in controlling movement. The normal functioning of the tendons relies on the nourishment of blood from the liver. If the liver is unable to supply the tendons adequately, spasm and atrophy of the limbs may result.

THE CONDITION OF THE LIVER CAN BE SEEN IN THE CONDITION OF THE NAILS.

The condition of the liver blood also influences the condition of the nails. When liver blood is sufficient, strong nails develop. When liver blood is deficient, the nails become thin and flexible, or even deformed. Thus, the condition of the liver can be determined by the condition of the nails.

THE LIVER IS LINKED TO THE EYES.

Because the liver stores blood and has channels linking it to the eyes, the liver plays an important role in the normal functioning of the eyes:

> When the liver is nourished by blood, good vision is preserved.
>> "Treatise on the Relationship between the
>> Outward Manifestation and the *Zang* Organs"
>> in *Plain Questions*
>
> Normal eyesight depends on the proper functioning of the liver because liver *qi* penetrates to the eyes.
>> "Treatise on the Length of Vessels"
>> in *Miraculous Pivot*

A deficiency of liver blood produces poor vision or night blindness. Further liver problems, such as an insufficiency of essence in the liver or the invasion of the Liver Channel by pathogenic wind-heat, can result in dryness of the eyes, in the former case, or conjunctivitis, in the latter.

THE LIVER AND GALLBLADDER FORM A *ZANG-FU* PAIR.

The gallbladder is attached to the liver and is a reservoir for bile. Bile, according to Chinese medicine, is a refined liquid formed by "the surplus liver *qi* that collects in the gallbladder," which is also known as the "reservoir of refined content." Together with the liver, the gallbladder helps promote the smooth flow of *qi* and blood.

The Spleen and the Stomach

> The spleen is the organ that stores intention and shares control of determination; with the heart, it decides everything.
>
> "Treatise on Acupuncture"
> in the *Addendum to Plain Questions*

> The spleen stores intention and governs thinking. Most importantly, it regulates the temperature of the body and moderates joy, anger, determination, and intention.
>
> Essentials of Confluent Traditional Chinese
> and Western Medicine

The spleen is located in the abdomen or middle burner. Together with the stomach, it is responsible for the digestion, assimilation, and distribution of nutrients and water throughout the body. Hence, the stomach and spleen are viewed as "the foundation of the latter heaven." That is, they form the material basis for the acquired constitution.[9] More specifically:

THE SPLEEN CONTROLS DIGESTION.

According to traditional Chinese medicine, nutrients are obtained from food by the combined digestive activities of the spleen and stomach. Nutrients are the essence of food, and this food essence is called "clarity." The spleen assimilates the nutrients, which are then conveyed throughout the body via the lung, heart, and vessels. This activity depends on spleen *qi,* which is said to "send clarity upward." That is, it transports the food essence to the lung and heart to be

---

9. See chapter 6, table 6.1, for an explanation of the Chinese distinction between the inherited and the acquired constitution.

disseminated through the body.[10] In addition to food essence, the spleen transmits water: water is absorbed first by the spleen and then transported along with the help of the lungs, heart, and urinary bladder to maintain normal water metabolism.

THE SPLEEN KEEPS BLOOD IN THE BLOOD VESSELS.

If spleen *qi* is sufficient, blood flows normally within the vessels. If it is not, then "blood can escape from the vessels." The resulting abnormalities include vaginal and subcutaneous bleeding.

THE SPLEEN STORES INTENTION.

Like the other *zang* organs, the spleen is involved in mental activities. It is said to store intention. Intention can be weakened by excessive mental strain. An impaired spleen results in mental turmoil, often marked by irritability, poor memory, and flaccid limbs.

THE SPLEEN CONTROLS THE LIMBS AND FLESH.

When the spleen functions normally, the body is adequately nourished; the muscles are well developed, and the limbs are strong. If the spleen's function is impeded, poor appetite results. A prolonged impairment of the spleen can lead to malnutrition, diarrhea, or edema due to retention of water. Hence, the flesh suffers.

THE SPLEEN IS LINKED TO THE MOUTH AND ITS CONDITION IS REFLECTED IN THE LIPS.

The mouth is linked most directly to the spleen. The connection is through the muscles, which the spleen nourishes. As a result of this connection, the condition of the spleen is reflected in the lips. Ruddy and lustrous lips signify that nutrients are being well assimilated. A malfunctioning of the spleen, on the other hand, causes an abnormal sense of taste, a poor appetite, and pale lips.

10. More recent scholars of traditional Chinese medicine assert that the spleen affects the secretory function of both the alimentary and respiratory systems, too. A deficiency of spleen *qi* has been observed to change the quality and quantity of the digestive fluids and to increase the secretion of phlegm. These observations are in concert with the traditional assertion that "the spleen is the source of phlegm."

THE SPLEEN AND STOMACH FORM A *ZANG-FU* PAIR.

The stomach has the function of taking in and digesting food into chyme. Just as the gallbladder is known as the reservoir for bile, the stomach is known as the reservoir for food and water. The forward movement of the partially digested food is regulated by stomach *qi*. Only when stomach *qi* is sufficient can the stomach carry out digestion and move the food on into the intestine for absorption. Thus:

> The vigor of the *zang-fu* organs is determined by the abundance of stomach *qi*, since the stomach is the important organ dominating digestion and the supply of nutrients.
>
> *The Treasured Classic*

The spleen and stomach work in coordination with each other, opposing yet complementing each other in order to accomplish the process of absorption and dissemination of nutrients. The spleen maintains the upward movement of *qi;* the stomach sends digested food downward. The spleen is said to have an aversion to dampness while the stomach prefers dampness.[11] Hence, the two organs work in harmony to guarantee a balanced process of digestion and absorption.[12]

The Lung and the Large Intestine

> *Qi* belongs to the lung.
>
> "Treatise on the Relationship between Outward Manifestations and the *Zang* Organs"
> in *Plain Questions*

11. One implication of this difference is that damp conditions, such as edema, are treated by strengthening the spleen, which will then work to eliminate the dampness.
Chinese clinical researchers also suggest that the spleen of Chinese medicine may accomplish some of the functions of the endocrine system of Western medicine. This suggestion is based on observations that patients suffering form chronic tracheitis of the "damp-phlegm" type (which results from deficient spleen *qi*) have a below normal plasma level of the hormone cortisol, and that a spleen tonic used specifically to treat damp-phlegm appears to affect the functioning of the adrenal cortex.
12. Many medical experts who have studied traditional Chinese medicine assert that the spleen, as described by Chinese medicine, corresponds to both the pancreas and spleen of Western medicine. However, based on guidelines for the differentiation of symptom-complexes in Chinese medicine (see chapter 8), it is clear that the spleen is more broadly involved in the activities of the digestive system than the spleen/pancreas of Western medicine; it is also an active part of the autonomic nervous system.

The lung is the organ responsible for respiration. It controls the inhaling of fresh air and the exhaling of spent air. But even more important, it governs the flow of *qi*. Thus, Chinese medicine describes it as follows:

THE LUNG CONTROLS *QI*.

The lung regulates the organs and tissues via pectoral *qi*, thereby controlling the body's essence and general *qi*. The general functioning of the organs therefore depends on the adequacy of lung *qi*. The lung also controls *wei qi*, which is defensive *qi*. Lung *qi* disperses *wei qi*, as well as body fluid, to all parts of the body to warm and nourish the skin and muscles. The skin, or surface layer of the body, is particularly dependent on the nourishment provided by the lung in the form of *wei qi* and body fluid. At the same time, the skin assists the lung in its functions. The sweat pore is known in Chinese medicine as the "portal of energy"; the opening and closing of these pores are governed by *wei qi*, which in turn is dependent on the lung's dispersing function. The skin thus assists in dispersing *wei qi* and in regulating respiration.

THE LUNG MAINTAINS THE DOWNWARD FLOW OF FLUID.

Lung *qi*, according to Chinese medicine, tends to flow downward. Water and fluids travel throughout the body and are discharged along routes or passageways that rely on this descending—and therefore cleansing—action of the lungs. Hence, the lung is said to maintain the flow of fluids, ensuring that they reach the urinary bladder. It helps maintain normal water metabolism. In fact, it is called "the upper source of water circulation." If this descending function of the lung is impeded, retention of fluids and edema occur.

THE LUNG STORES VITALITY.

Vitality is a mental activity and is closely related to *qi:*

> *Qi*, which is stored in the lung, holds vitality.
>
> "Treatise on Mental and Life Activities"
> in *Miraculous Pivot*

Vitality can be seen in a person who is fully absorbed in what he or she is doing; such a person usually breathes evenly and gently and performs his or her work with boldness and resolution. Persistent sorrow and anxiety can lead to the stagnation and obstruction of lung *qi*. The result is likely to be dejection, irritability, depression, and hesitance, all of which suggest that vitality has been impaired.

THE LUNG IS LINKED TO THE NOSE.

The nose is part of the passageway of the respiratory system. A keen sense of smell, as well as normal respiration, depend on the smooth flow of lung *qi*. Thus:

> A normal nose is able to differentiate a sweet smell from a foul smell because lung *qi* permeates the nose.
>
> > "Treatise on the Length of the Vessels,"
> > in the *Miraculous Pivot*

THE LUNG AND THE LARGE INTESTINE FORM A *ZANG-FU* PAIR.

The external organ associated with the lung is the large intestine. The functions of the large intestine, like those of other *fu* organs, are to "convey" and "transform." In the large intestine, unusable material from the small intestine is transformed into solid wastes as the water is absorbed; these are then expelled from the body. Chinese medicine therefore states that "The large intestine governs body fluid."

As in all *zang-fu* pairs, the lung and large intestine cooperate in their physiological functions and affect each other when diseased. When the descending function of the lung *qi* is normal, the large intestine functions efficiently, and elimination occurs freely. When this function is not normal, obstruction of the large intestine can occur. Conversely, if the large intestine is obstructed, the descending function of lung *qi* may be blocked.[13]

13. One approach to understanding the lung of traditional Chinese medicine in Western terms has been to study *"qigong."* Qigong is a system of breathing exercise therapy; studies of this system indicate that the lung is the only organ that is under both voluntary and involuntary control. Because of the connections between the lung and other systems not normally associated with the lung in Western medicine, exercises such as *qigong* offer the potential of voluntarily controlling systems not normally under voluntary control. For example, *qigong* can have beneficial effects on the autonomic nervous system, digestion, circulation, metabolism, and reproduction.

The Kidney and the Urinary Bladder

The kidney takes in and stores the essence of the *zang-fu* organs.
"Treatise on Natural Essence in Ancient Times"
in *Plain Questions*

According to Chinese medicine, the kidney promotes the growth and development of the body and helps control reproduction, water metabolism, and respiration. More specifically, it performs the following functions:

THE KIDNEY STORES VITAL ESSENCE AND VITAL FUNCTION.

The kidney stores genuine *yin* and *yang* or vital essence and vital function.[14] Vital essence is the material basis of life. It is composed of two parts: reproductive essence, which controls reproduction; and the essence of the *zang-fu* organs,[15] which controls growth, development, and other life activities. The first of these is acquired from one's parents; the second is produced by the spleen and stomach. Both are stored in the kidney.

The reproductive or congenital essence is the material basis of the embryo and is the essential factor for growth following birth. When a person has matured, his kidney essence becomes rich; kidney *qi* is abundant; and the reproductive organs are fully developed. At this time, the male is capable of secreting sperm, and the female menstruates.

Part of the acquired essence of the *zang-fu* organs is used to satisfy the demands of organs and tissues for their vital activities, but the remaining portion is stored in the kidney to be used for the growth and development of the body. Chinese medicine explains that this kidney essence can be transformed into *qi,* known as kidney *qi*. The rise and fall of kidney *qi* then influences reproduction, growth, and development.

Chinese medicine speaks of a "vital gate," which is viewed as the

14. Genuine *yin* and *yang* is derived from one's parents. It is the basis of the inherited (as opposed to the acquired) constitution and is known as the "source of the former heaven." (See chapter 6, table 6.1.)

15. Reproductive essence is also known as "essence of the former heaven"; the essence of the *zang-fu* organs is also known as "essence of the latter heaven."

source of life. The "fire" or source of energy of the vital gate is kidney *yang* (or genuine *yang*). This is the dynamic force of reproduction and development as well as the source of the *yang qi* for all the other organs.[16]

THE KIDNEY PRODUCES MARROW.

The vital essence stored by the kidney forms bone marrow. The bones, in turn, grow strong when they are properly nourished by the marrow. Marrow is of two types: bone marrow and the spinal marrow that permeates the brain. Chinese medicine asserts that the brain is formed of marrow and hence calls it the "reservoir of marrow." Since marrow is formed out of vital essence from the kidney, the brain is closely connected with the kidney.

THE KIDNEY REGULATES WATER IN THE BODY.

The balance of water in the body depends on the normal activity of the kidney. Body fluid is of two types: "clear fluid" circulates throughout the organs, tissues, and muscles, while the "turbid fluid" is transformed into sweat and urine to be discharged from the body. For the proper balance of water in the body, both of these activities are necessary. The kidney has the ability to transport the clear fluid upward, to discharge the turbid fluid downward, and to reabsorb fluids in large quantities. In this way, the kidney regulates water circulation. Any failure of the kidney leads to disturbances in water metabolism, accompanied by inability to urinate, edema, and similar symptoms.

THE KIDNEY HELPS COORDINATE RESPIRATION.

The kidney also plays a role in respiration. Though controlled by the lung, respiration is coordinated by the kidney during inhalation.

---

16. The function of the fire of the vital gate is similar to the action of parts of the endocrine system of Western medicine, including the functions of the adrenals, sex glands, and the pituitary. Autopsies of patients who have been diagnosed as having deficiency of kidney *yang* reveal changes in morphology indicative of hypofunctioning of endocrine glands, including the adrenal, thyroid, and testis. Postmortem examinations of patients who had shown no deficiency symptom-complex for the kidney did not reveal any such changes.

By directing *qi* downward, the kidney aids the lung in inhaling. When kidney *qi* is abundant and inhalation is normal, the passageway for *qi* is clear; breathing is even. If the kidney fails to maintain normal inhalation, asthma of the "deficiency type"[17] may appear. This type of asthma is characterized by increased exhalation and decreased inhalation.

THE KIDNEY STORES DETERMINATION.

Generally, when kidney *qi* is abundant, an individual will demonstrate determination; abundant kidney *qi* produces rich essence and marrow, resulting in good memory, vigor, wisdom, and well-developed skills. However, when kidney *qi* is weak, such clinical symptoms as poor memory, low spirits, a lack of aspiration, and premature senility may all appear.

Also, extreme anger or terror may impair the kidney and thus impair determination. Since the kidney nourishes the brain—especially the function of memory storage—temporary amnesia may result in such cases.

THE CONDITION OF THE KIDNEY CAN BE SEEN IN THE CONDITION OF THE HAIR.

The hair on one's head depends on kidney *qi* for its vitality.[18] Nourished by blood, hair is known as "the extension of blood." Blood, in turn, is related to vital essence; the two are said to be interpromoting and intertransforming. Rich essence stored in the kidney yields abundant blood, which nourishes the hair. Accordingly, Chinese medicine states that the condition of the kidney can be judged from the hair and that the adequacy of kidney essence or *qi* can be seen in the growth, lustre, and loss of hair.

THE KIDNEY IS LINKED TO THE EARS, THE GENITALS, AND THE ANUS.

The kidney is connected by channels to three body orifices: the ears, the genitals, and the anus. Hearing thus depends on kidney

17. See chapter 8 for a classification of deficiency and excess syndromes.
18. Body hair is distinct from the hair on one's head; body hair is nourished by lung *qi* rather than kidney *qi*.

qi.[19] Reproduction is also governed by kidney *qi;* hence, the connection with the genitals. Finally, the kidney promotes the discharge of urine through the genitals and the elimination of wastes through the anus.

THE KIDNEY AND THE URINARY BLADDER FORM A ZANG-FU PAIR.

The kidney's *fu* organ is the urinary bladder, which temporarily stores and then discharges urine. As already explained, the kidney separates usable (or clear) fluid from unusable (or turbid) fluid. The latter flow into the urinary bladder to be discharged from the body. This function of the bladder is directed by the *yang* activity of the kidney.

PROMOTING, RESTRAINING, BALANCE, AND HARMONIZING: THE RELATIONSHIP AMONG ZANG ORGANS

> A disorder of the mother element affects the son element; a disorder of the son element affects the mother element.
>
> "The Sixty-ninth Problem"
> in *Classic on Medical Problems*

Just as the *zang-fu* organs interact in pairs, so do the *zang* organs interact with one another.[20] The relationship between the *zang* and *fu* organs is governed by the principles of *yin* and *yang;* the relationships among the *zang* organs is governed by the principles of the five-element theory. These relationships may be summarized as follows:

THE HEART AND THE LUNG. The heart governs blood, and the lung controls *qi.* Both organs work in coordination to control the circulation of blood. Sufficient blood produces abundant lung *qi,* which, in turn, ensures normal circulation. If lung *qi* becomes insufficient,

19. According to the "Treatise on the Length of Vessels" in *Miraculous Pivot:* "The kidney is associated with the ear. A normal kidney therefore guarantees a good sense of hearing."

20. Less significant, but still important, is the relationship among the *fu* organs. This involves coordinating the process of digestion, absorption, and elimination. Lack of coordination of the *fu* organs typically leads to digestive and eliminatory disorders.

circulation is impaired, and the resulting decline in the heart's functioning impedes respiration.

THE HEART AND THE KIDNEY. The heart corresponds to fire; it is located in the upper burner. The kidney corresponds to water and is in the lower burner. The relationship between the two is the "harmonious relationship between water and fire." They balance each other, each assisting and checking the action of the other. If this balance breaks down, symptoms such as restlessness, insomnia, vertigo, ringing in the ears, muscular aching, and a sensation of weakness in the lumbar region or knee joints may occur. These symptoms are referred to in Chinese medicine as "the discord of the heart and kidney."

THE HEART AND THE LIVER. The heart governs the entire cardiovascular system, while the liver stores and regulates blood. An abundance of blood allows the heart and liver to work efficiently. An insufficiency of blood and a deficiency of liver *qi* produces a set of symptoms described as "the failure of blood to nourish the muscles and tendons." Such symptoms include numbness and aching in the bones and muscles as well as spasms. The heart and liver also cooperate in regulating mental activities, which depend not only on the functioning of the heart, but also on the smooth flow of *qi,* governed by the liver.

THE HEART AND THE SPLEEN. The heart governs the blood, which is produced by the spleen. An abundance of spleen *qi* is the basis for growth and transformation of blood. Thus, normal blood circulation in the vessels relies not only on the promoting action of heart *qi,* but also on the controlling action of spleen *qi*. For this reason, the growth and circulation of blood is an indicator of how well the heart and spleen are working together.

THE LUNG AND THE SPLEEN. Food essence that is transformed by the spleen supplies the lung with *qi*. In turn, the dispersing and descending function of lung *qi* helps the spleen in its transport and transformation of water. A deficiency of lung *qi* can thus sometimes be treated not only by medicines that invigorate the lung, but also by those that invigorate the spleen.

THE LUNG AND THE LIVER. The relationship between the liver and the lung is based on the ascending and descending movements of *qi*. The lung dominates the descending action of *qi* and can thus balance the tendency of liver *qi* to rise. For this reason, Chinese medicine says that "lung-metal restrains liver-wood." If the balance is upset and the lung is invaded by excessive liver heat, the result is a condition described as "wood-fire causing metal to suffer." Some of the symptoms of this condition include irritability, gastric pain, and cough, accompanied by dyspepsia and coughing up of blood.

THE LUNG AND THE KIDNEY. The lung and kidney are related through their mutual control of *qi* and water. The lung controls *qi,* but the kidney promotes the inhalation that is a necessary part of the functioning of the lung. Therefore, in Chinese medicine, the lung is known as the "mother of *qi*" while the kidney is the "foundation of *qi*." Regarding water, the kidney regulates its circulation while the lung is its upper source. Water metabolism thus also depends on both the kidney and the lung.

THE SPLEEN AND THE LIVER. The ascending, descending, transporting, and transforming actions of the spleen and stomach depend on the liver's ability to ensure the smooth flow of *qi*. Either an overabundant liver *qi* or a weak spleen *qi* can create a condition known as "liver-wood encroaching on the spleen." This is a discord between the liver and the spleen or between the liver and the stomach. Symptoms of this condition are pain in the costal and epigastric regions, abdominal distension, and abnormal bowel movements, among others.

THE SPLEEN AND THE KIDNEY. The spleen provides the material basis of the acquired constitution while the kidney is the storehouse of the native constitution. The function of the spleen is to digest food and to transform and disseminate nutrients. In order to carry out this function, the spleen depends on kidney *yang*—on the "fire of the vital gate." In turn, kidney essence constantly needs to be replenished by the nutrients supplied by the spleen. These two organs, then, promote and aid each other in their functions. When one is diseased, the other may easily become diseased also; symptom-complexes involving a deficiency of both kidney and spleen are common.

THE LIVER AND THE KIDNEY. Liver blood is nourished by kidney essence. Chinese medicine states that "essence and blood have a common source" or that "the liver and kidney have a common source." The overconsumption of kidney *yin* often leads to insufficient liver *yin*. This deficiency results in the failure of *yin* to restrain *yang* in the two organs. An intensification of liver *yang,* in turn, produces dizziness and high blood pressure.

THE MISCELLANEOUS ORGANS: ORGANS OF CONSCIOUSNESS

In addition to the *zang* and *fu* organs, traditional Chinese medicine recognizes several organs that do not fit into either of these two basic classes. They call these simply "miscellaneous" organs. They include the brain, bone, bone marrow, blood vessels, the uterus, and the gallbladder. (The gallbladder is considered to be both a *fu* organ and a miscellaneous organ. It is the former because it is hollow in structure. But because the bile stored in the gallbladder is not waste to be excreted, the gallbladder is also known as a miscellaneous organ.)

The miscellaneous organs have characteristics of both the *zang* and the *fu* organs. They are hollow and thus resemble the *fu* organs in shape. But they are also organs of storage:

> These six organs, similar to the earth and thus pertaining to yin, are capable of storing without discharging because they are nourished by the earth, which is considered the mother of many things.
>
> "Further Discussions of the *Zang* Organs"
> in *Plain Questions*

The miscellaneous organs store essence. Since essence is the material basis for consciousness, their functions are all related to consciousness. The brain is the source of "mentalilty." The blood vessels house this mentality. The gallbladder, located in the center of the body, governs decision-making. The bone is the source of the marrow, which is considered a continuation of the brain. The uterus is where new consciousness (that is, new life) develops.

ORIGINS OF THE THEORY OF THE ZANG-FU ORGANS

Anatomy was part of the study of traditional Chinese medicine as long ago as the appearance of the *Classic of Internal Medicine.* This volume not only describes the internal organs; it also explains the formation, nature, and function of blood and the vessels. In addition, it describes the source of circulation, the parts of the organs to which the blood travels, and the rate at which it travels. A detailed description of the shapes of organs as observed during human dissections appears as follows:

> A man's skin and flesh can be measured on the surface of the body and his organs' sizes felt by palpation. Also, when a man is dead, his organs can be observed by autopsy. The good, bad condition of the *zang* and the size of the *fu* organs; the amount of nutrients they absorb; the length of the vessels; the condition of the blood; the amount of *qi;* all of these can be defined.
>
> "Treatise on the Comparison of Channels
> to Rivers" in *Miraculous Pivot*

Another example indicates the level of knowledge of anatomical measurements:

> It (the gastrointestinal tract) is one *chi* (*chi* = ⅓ meter) and six *cun* (*cun* = ⅓ decimeter) from the pharynx to the convoluted stomach; if the stomach is stretched, its length is two *chi* and six *cun*. . . . The total length from the opening of the stomach to the end of the intestines is six *zhang* (*zhang* = ⅓ meters), four *cun* and four *fen* (*fen* = ⅓ centimeter).
>
> "Treatise on the Intestines and Stomach"
> in *Miraculous Pivot*

Though the unit length in the Qin dynasty (221–207 B.C.) is smaller than that of today, the ratio of the length of the esophagus to the length of the large and small intestines combined is 1:35, which approximates the present known value. The length of various portions of the body, as well as the shape, linear measurement, and volume of the alimentary tract and various organs are also recorded in such classics as the "Treatise on Fasting" in *Miraculous Pivot* and in the *Classic on Medical Problems.*

More important than determining the shape and size of the various parts of the body was the goal of understanding the functions of these parts and their relationship to each other. To accomplish this goal, the ancient Chinese studied the differing reactions of the human body to changing external conditions. The configuration of the body, the internal organs, the channels, acupoints, muscles, joints, bones, tissues and their activities, as well as their interaction with the external environment were deduced from such observations.

The common cold provides a simple example of this process. A cold is accompanied by symptoms of a stuffy nose, nasal discharge, and cough. This set of symptoms told the ancient Chinese observer that the nose is specifically related to the lungs.

Similarly, those with a weak constitution and an aversion to wind perspire more and are more susceptible to illness than those who are healthy. From this observation, the early Chinese practitioners concluded that *"wei qi"* (or the defensive function of the human body) is disseminated on the surface of the skin; it "warms the muscles, nourishes the tissues, and controls the opening and closing of the pores," guarding against pathogens.

Another example comes from the observation that mental anxiety often produces a poor appetite and dyspepsia. Long-term observation of this correlation led the ancient Chinese to connect mental activity to the digestive and absorptive functions of the spleen. Hence, the *zang-fu* theory states that "the spleen governs thinking; mental anxiety impairs the spleen."

Finally, traditional Chinese medicine has had a long clinical history, during which inferences about the *zang-fu* organs have been made by correlating symptoms with the results of specific treatments. For example, it was observed that the symptoms of chills, fever, coughing, and wheezing could be treated successfully with medicines that disperse *qi* and induce perspiration. From such observations came the argument that the lungs are connected with the skin and that an adverse flow of lung *qi* causes coughing.

The connection between the liver and emotional depression was inferred from the observation that emotional depression readily causes gastric pain, an oppressed sensation in the chest, and frequent sighing. Traditional Chinese physicians found that they could relieve these symptoms by restoring the normal functioning of a depressed liver. Traditional medicine therefore asserts that the liver governs the smooth flow of *qi* and is unfavorably affected by depression.

Chinese medicine also says that "the spleen nourishes the limbs and muscles." This conclusion evolved from repeated observation that those who suffer from feeble limbs, a gaunt form, and swollen muscles could be treated by using methods to reinforce the functioning of the spleen and to dispel dampness. Chinese practitioners concluded that these symptoms are the result of hypofunctioning of the spleen and stomach, which affect digestion and absorption. This condition may be accompanied by the invasion of "pathogenic dampness"; hence methods that dispel dampness are necessary.

As a final example, many kidney tonics were observed to speed the healing of bone fractures. Chinese physicians thus concluded that the vital essence of the kidney promotes the repair and growth of bones.

IN SUMMARY

Traditional Chinese medicine describes the activities of the body in terms of the *zang-fu* organs.

There are five *zang* organs: the heart, liver, spleen, lung, and kidney. They are characterized as solid organs and are said to be *yin* in nature. Corresponding to the five *zang* organs are the six *fu* organs: the gallbladder, stomach, small intestine, large intestine, urinary bladder and Triple Burner. These are the hollow organs and are said to be *yang* in nature. The *zang* organs are organs of storage. The *fu* organs are organs of transfer; they do not store materials. In addition to the *zang* and *fu* organs are the so-called "miscellaneous" organs; the brain, blood vessels, bone, bone marrow, gallbladder, and uterus. These organs function as organs of both storage and transfer and are specifically related to consciousness.

The *zang-fu* organs interact with each other in pairs. The activities of each *zang* organ depend on those of the corresponding *fu* organ, and vice-versa. Similarly, if one member of a *zang-fu* pair fails to function properly, the other will also become diseased.

The *zang* organs also interact with one another, following the basic pattern of relationships described by the theory of the five elements.

In the theory of the *zang-fu* organs, the concept of an organ is different from that in Western medicine. Rather than a single anatomical structure, the organ of traditional Chinese medicine is a system of structures and tissues that form an energy network through the body. The principal pathways of these energy networks are known as channels; they are described in detail in chapter 4.

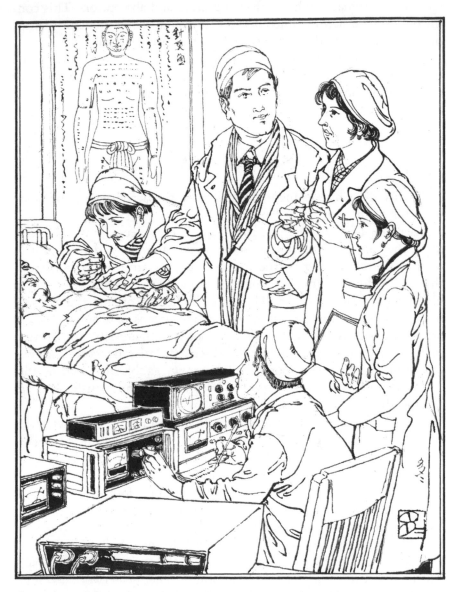

Acupuncturists and scientists using modern technology to study channels and collaterals.

CHAPTER FOUR

The Channel System

We must have a deep understanding of the channels because, through them, life and death can be judged, diseases diagnosed, deficiency and excess regulated.

"Treatise on the Channels and Collaterals" in
Miraculous Pivot

TOGETHER WITH THE theory of the *zang-fu* organs, the theory of the channel system constitutes the anatomy of traditional Chinese medicine. The channel system is a system of pathways throughout the body. However, just as the *zang-fu* organs are not strictly analogous to the concrete organs that bear the same names in Western medicine, the channels of Chinese medicine are not analogous to any tangible channel in the human body, such as the veins and arteries. Rather, they are a way of describing the flow of blood, *qi* (or vital energy), and information that supports the life functions of the body. In this sense, they are more invisible than visible.

In addition to its description of the anatomy of the human body, the theory of the channel system helps explain pathology and the course of disease. It also forms the basis for both a theory of treatment and a variety of clinical practices. In the West, the best known of these clinical practices is acupuncture, which seeks to tonify and disperse *qi* by physically stimulating points along the pathways that convey it. However, the concept of the channel system has also been adopted as a basis for other forms of therapies, including herbal medicine. It is thus a major component of traditional Chinese medicine.

THE CHANNEL SYSTEM: COMMUNICATION, REGULATION, AND DISTRIBUTION

Internally, the twelve channels are connected with the *zang-fu* organs; externally, with the extremities and their joints.

"Treatise on the Seas"
in *Miraculous Pivot*

Their function is to make *qi* and blood flow. Through them, the tendons and bones are moistened; the joints become nimble because *yin* and *yang* are in harmony. The smooth travel of *qi* and blood in the channels brings nutrients to the body, helps the balance of *yin* and *yang*, invigorates the tendons, bones, and joints.

"Treatise on the Original Organs"
in *Miraculous Pivot*

The channel system of the body serves three major functions. The first is communication. Since the body is an organic whole, all of its parts—the *zang* and *fu* organs, the extremities and bones, the five sense organs, the nine orifices, and the flesh, muscles, and vessels— must work harmoniously to carry out the processes of life, even though each has its own individual physiological action. This harmonious functioning of the body depends on the ability of its parts to communicate with one another.

The channel system provides this means of communication. It forms a network for communication between the internal organs and the extremities. It connects the upper and the lower as well as the interior and exterior parts of the body. In this way, it is possible for the internal organs to remain responsive to the conditions that the body encounters in the environment.

The second function of the channels is the *regulation* or coordination of the activities of the *zang* and *fu* organs. As described in the previous chapter, the pairs of *zang-fu* organs are interrelated in their functioning. They support and restrain each other. The orderly flow of *qi* through the channels is the means through which this mutual regulation occurs.

The third major function of the channel system is *distribution*. The channels may be viewed as passageways in which *qi* and blood flow.[1]

---

1. The channels of traditional Chinese medicine are *not* analogous to the blood vessels of Western medicine. They are energy pathways through the body, and blood along with other life substances just happens to be there.

This circulatory function ensures that the tissues and organs in all parts of the body are supplied with nutrients and fluids. The motivating force that promotes this circulation is called "channel *qi*" (or the vital energy of the channels). Channel *qi* is, in turn, a mirror of channel activity, and ultimately of the activity of the *zang-fu* organs.

Because it is the means of communication, regulation, and distribution of vital substances throughout the body, the channel system is also the route that pathological changes follow between the *zang* and *fu* organs and between the internal organ structures and the superficial tissues. The onset of a disease in the internal organs will thus ultimately find expression in a given location on the exterior of the body.

THE CHANNELS: AN ANATOMY OF THE HUMAN BODY

The theory of the channel system, in its simplest form, describes the human body as analogous to three concentric cylinders. The innermost cylinder houses the internal organs. The second cylinder houses the principal channels of the channel system. The third, or outermost cylinder, is the surface layer of the body; it is permeated by branches of the channel system that communicate between the surface of the body and the channels. Within this overall pattern of organization are seven different kinds of channels, each with a distinct function.

The Twelve Principal Channels

The main trunks of the channel system are the Twelve Principal Channels. These channels run lengthwise through the body in what can be imagined as the middle cylinder. Each channel is associated with either a *zang* or a *fu* organ. Those that are associated with *zang* organs are the *yin* channels. Those associated with the *fu* organs are the *yang* channels. Also, each *yang* channel has a secondary relationship with a *zang* organ; such channels are said to *communicate* with the *zang* organs. Similarly, each *yin* channel has a secondary relationship—and therefore communicates—with a *fu* organ. The *yin* channels, being associated with the *zang* organs, convey the interior energy of the body, while the *yang* channels convey the more exterior energy.

The Twelve Principal Channels also divide the task of communicating with the upper and lower parts of the body. Six of them
communicate with the lower half of the body, passing through the
legs and feet; these are known as the "Foot Channels." The remaining six travel through the upper half of the body, passing through
the arms and hands; they are known as the "Hand Channels." The
yin channels are located on the medial (or inner) side of the extremities, while the *yang* are located on the lateral (or outer) side.

One more set of distinctions is important in differentiating the
Twelve Principal Channels. The various Hand and Foot Channels
follow different pathways along the extremities. These pathways are
distinguished as follows:

— Those Hand and Food Channels that are located on the *front* side
of the extremities are known as the Channels of *Taiyin* and
Yangming.[2]
— Those that are located on the *back* side of the extremities are
known as the channels of *Shaoyin* and *Taiyang*.
— Those that are located *midway* between the front and the back of
the extremities are known as the channels of *Jueyin* and *Shaoyang*.

TABLE 4.1. Summary of the Twelve Principal Channels

Location		Yin *Channel* (medial side)	Yang *Channel* (lateral side)
Hand channel (upper extremities)	Front	Lung Channel of hand-taiyin	Large Intestine Channel of hand-yangming
	Midway	Pericardium Channel of hand-jueyin	Triple Burner Channel of hand-shaoyang
	Back	Heart Channel of hand-shaoyin	Small Intestine Channel of hand-taiyang
Foot channel (lower extremities)	Front	Spleen Channel of foot-taiyin	Stomach Channel of foot-yangming
	Midway	Liver Channel of foot-jueyin	Gallbladder Channel of foot-shaoyang
	Back	Kidney Channel of foot-shaoyin	Urinary Bladder Channel of foot-taiyang

2. These locations refer to the position of the arms as they hang at one's side with palms
facing inwards.

All of these distinctions are summarized in the names of the Twelve Principal Channels, as shown in table 4.1.

Each of the Twelve Principal Channels travels in a fixed direction. The direction of flow is as follows:

—The three *yin* channels of the hand start in the chest and flow to the hand, where they meet the three *yang* channels of the hand.

—The three *yang* channels of the hand start from the hand and ascend to the head, where they meet the three *yang* channels of the foot.

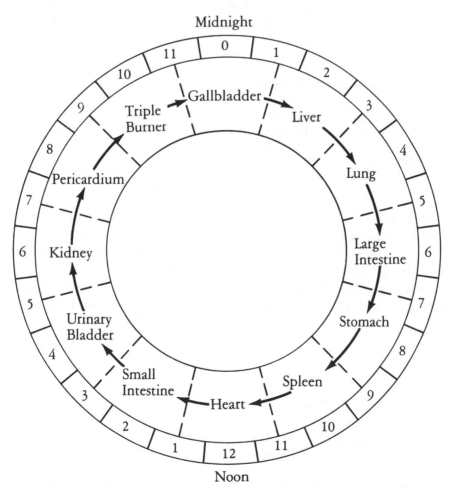

FIGURE 4.1. Daily Cycle of *Qi* through the Twelve Principal Channels

—The three *yang* channels of the foot start from the head, run
toward the foot, and there meet the three *yin* channels of the
foot.
—The three *yin* channels of the foot start from the foot, ascend to
the abdomen, and meet the three *yin* channels of the hand.

Each channel meets another channel. At the point where they meet,
there is a transfer of channel *qi*. In this way, the Twelve Principal
Channels guarantee the orderly flow of *qi* throughout the body. This
flow of *qi* creates a cycle. Each cycle lasts 24 hours. That is, the
"peak" of *qi* flow is in each of the channels for two hours each day.
Through this cycle, the continuous flow of *qi* throughout the body
is guaranteed. (See figure 4.1).

The Eight Extra Channels

> There are two kinds of channels, extra and regular. The Twelve Principal
> Channels are the regular whereas the Eight Extra Channels are not—they
> are known as extraordinary ones. *Qi* and blood circulate in the Twelve
> Channels of the human body. They flow into the Eight Extra Channels if
> the former become overfilled.
>
> *General Collection for Holy Relief*

The second group of channels is the Eight Extra Channels. They
differ from the Twelve Principal Channels in two ways: they are not
directly related to any of the internal organs nor are they related to
one another in an interior/exterior relationship.[3]
The Eight Extra Channels are interlaced with the Twelve Principal
Channels and help to reinforce the communication between pairs of
them. They help assure a steady flow of *qi* and blood, accommodat-
ing an overflow when a surplus exists and replenishing a channel
when *qi* and blood are insufficient.

The Divergent Channels

The Divergent Channels supplement the Twelve Principal Channels, enhancing communication along the *yin* and *yang* channels and

3. The Eight Extra Channels are sometimes described as "primordial." That is, they are
the source of development of the rest of the body.

among the internal organs, and ensuring close coordination between the exterior and interior of the body.

They branch from the Twelve Principal Channels, usually at the extremities. They then follow a course that approximately parallels the Twelve Principal Channels, creating another concentric cylinder. In this way, they strengthen the transmission of stimulus from the outside to the inside. They also establish stronger ties between the Twelve Principal Channels and the head, since the six *yin* channels do not run to the head, while the Divergent Channels do.

Each Divergent Channel is associated with a pair of principal channels. The courses of the Divergent Channels can thus be classified into six groups based on their *yin* and *yang* relationships as well as their internal and external relationship (in the same way as the Twelve Principal Channels are classified in table 4.1). The *yang* Divergent Channels arise from the six *yang* Principal Channels at the body surface. They then separate and travel to their respective *fu* organs. Later, they reemerge at the nape of the neck and once again combine with the six *yang* Principal Channels. The *yin* Channels follow a similar course, but they finally also combine with the six *yang* Principal Channels. This course is known as the "six combinations."

Finally, the Divergent Channels strengthen the connection between the three hand-*yin* and three hand-*yang* channels, and between the three foot-*yin* and three foot-*yang* channels, or essentially between the internal channels of the *zang*-organs and the external channels of the *fu*-organs.

The Connecting Channels

The Connecting Channels are actually branches that diverge from the Twelve Principal Channels and the Eight Extra Channels. There are fifteen of them, and their principal task is to maintain communication between the neighboring channels.

The Tendon/Muscle Channels

In the picture of the body as three concentric cylinders, the outermost cylinder houses a system of flesh and joints that form a series of channels known as the Tendon/Muscle Channels. These are areas where the *qi* of the Twelve Principal Channels gathers, joins, disperses, and connects. Because the Tendon/Muscle Channels are located in the superficial tissues, they mainly affect the muscles and tendons. They do not enter the internal organs, and when they are diseased, they usually produce symptoms in the muscles of the extremities, head, and trunk rather than in the internal organs.

These channels are not in an internal/external relationship and hence do not circulate in a circular course. They are, however, divided in the same way as the principal channels into pairs of three *yin* and three *yang* channels for both the feet and the hands.

The Tendon/Muscle Channels follow a course quite different from that of the Twelve Principal Channels, and, in fact, they reach parts of the body that the principal channels fail to reach. Thus, they not only carry the flow of energy along the surface of the body; they also supplement the Twelve Principal Channels.

The Cutaneous Regions of the Twelve Principal Channels

In certain areas of the skin, the functioning of the Twelve Principal Channels can be seen. These areas are thus included in the description of the channel system. They are places where pathogenic factors from the external environment may enter the body. Also, diseases in the interior of the body will produce characteristic signs in these skin regions. Accordingly, they are often the points at which external energy, in the form of treatments such as acupuncture and massage, can be introduced into the channel system. (These are not, however, the sole points for treatment.)

Superficial and Tertiary Channels

Finally, there are countless small collateral channels distributed throughout the body. These superficial channels, as their name suggests, have their courses along the surface of the body. The smallest of the channels—the tertiary collaterals—form a complex of passages for blood and *qi* to circulate between the interior and exterior channels.

THE COURSE OF THE CHANNELS

A knowledge of the specific course of each channel through the body is essential both in diagnosing and in treating disease. This course has two parts—a surface part and a deep part—allowing the channel to function in its role of connecting the body surface to the internal organs. Along the surface are many points where the energy of the channel can be treated by the practitioners. These points are numbered sequentially for each channel, thereby tracking its surface path. The diagrams accompanying the descriptions of the channel courses illustrate these paths and points.

Abbreviations for the channels used in naming the points are as follows:

Lu — Lung	UB — Urinary Bladder
LI — Large Intestine	K — Kidney
St — Stomach	P — Pericardium
Sp — Spleen	SJ — Triple Burner
H — Heart	GB — Gall Bladder
SI — Small Intestine	Liv — Liver

This nomenclature is based on *The Essentials of Chinese Acupuncture* (Beijing: Foreign Languages Press, 1980).

The Twelve Principal Channels

THE LUNG CHANNEL OF HAND-TAIYIN (FIGURE 4.2)

- The Lung Channel of Hand-Taiyin originates in the middle burner.
- It descends to connect with the large intestine.
- It swings back up following the cardiac orifice.
- It passes through the diaphragm to enter the lung.
- It ascends the trachea to the throat.
- It exits transversely to the exterosuperior region of the chest.
- It descends along the medial side of the arms.
- It passes the *"cun kou"* point above the radial artery of the wrist where the pulse is felt.
- It branches, with one branch descending to the tip of the thumb.
- The other branch separates at the back of the wrist and runs di-

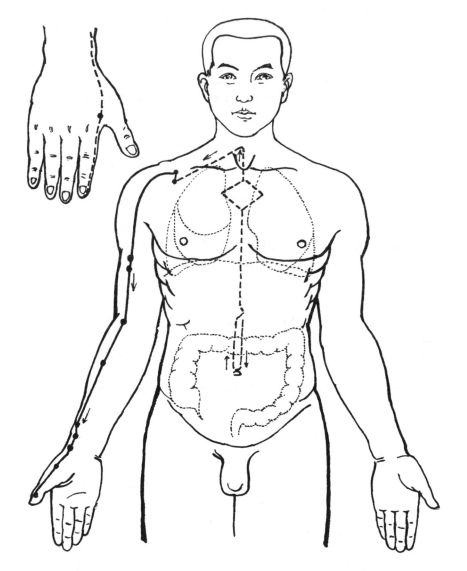

FIGURE 4.2.   Lung Channel of Hand-Taiyin

rectly along the lateral side of the dorsum of the hand to the
radial side of the index finger.

- It connects with the Large Intestine Channel of Hand-Yangming
  at Shangyang point (LI 1).

THE LARGE INTESTINE CHANNEL OF HAND-YANGMING (FIGURE 4.3)

- The Large Intestine Channel of Hand-Yangming starts from the
  tip of the index finger.
- It runs along the interior border of the lateral side of the upper
  extremities.
- It goes up to the highest point of the shoulder.
- It passes the seventh cervical vertebra.
- It descends into the supraclavicular fossa.
- It divides into two branches.
- The first branch enters the chest to the lung, and then runs
  downward through the diaphragm to connect with the large in-
  testine.
- The second branch ascends through the neck and cheek and en-
  ters the lower teeth and gum.
- The second branch continues to curve around the upper lip,
  crossing the other channel of Hand-Yangming and traveling to
  the side of the nostril.
- It connects with the Stomach Channel of Foot-Yangming at
  Yingxiang point (LI 20).

THE STOMACH CHANNEL OF FOOT-YANGMING (FIGURE 4.4)

- The Stomach Channel of Foot-Yangming starts at the side of the
  nostril.
- It travels upward and intersects the bridge of the nose.
- It enters the inner canthus laterally, communicating with the
  Urinary Bladder Channel of Foot-Taiyang.
- It descends along the orbit of the eye and enters the upper gum.
- It emerges from the gum and curves around the lips.
- It meets the Ren Channel in the center of the lower jaw at
  Cheng-jiang point (Ren 24).
- It turns back, traveling in front of the ear and along the side of
  the forehead.

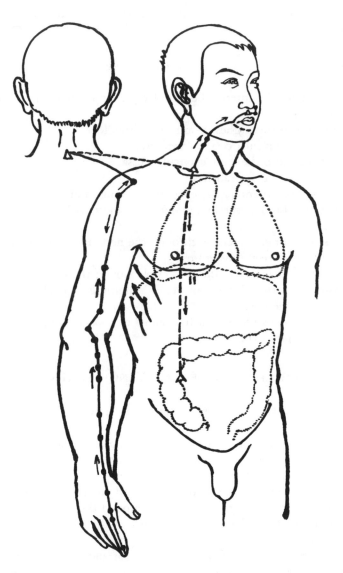

FIGURE 4.3.   Large Intestine Channel of Hand-Yangming

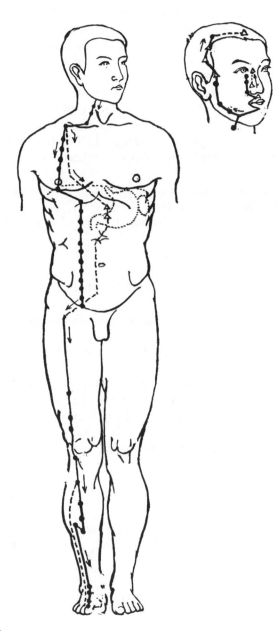

FIGURE 4.4. Stomach Channel of Foot-Yangming

- It descends from the cheek, traveling laterally along the throat to the supraclavicular fossa.
- It divides into two branches.
- The first branch descends through the chest and diaphragm to the stomach, spleen, and on toward the groin.
- The second branch descends laterally on the body surface along the mamillary line, 2 *cun*[4] to the side of the umbilicus and down to the groin.
- It merges with the first branch at the groin.
- It descends along the lateral side of the leg to the dorsum of the foot, reaching the lateral side of the tip of the second toe.
- Two other branches appear in the leg; the first begins at the posterior edge of the patella and ends at the lateral side of the middle toe.
- The other branch splits from the dorsum of the foot and terminates at the medial side of the big toe.
- This branch connects with the Spleen Channel of Foot-Taiyin at Yinbai point (Sp 1).

THE SPLEEN CHANNEL OF FOOT-TAIYIN (FIGURE 4.5)

- The Spleen Channel of Foot-Taiyin originates on the medial side of the big toe.
- It passes along the medial side of the foot at the juncture of the so-called "red and white" skin.[5]
- It ascends in front of the medial malleolus up the leg.
- It follows the posterior side of the tibia to a point 8 *cun* above the inner malleolus, where it crosses in front of the Liver Channel of Foot-Jueyin.
- It ascends along the front of the medial side of the thigh.
- It enters the abdomen to the spleen and stomach
- The first branch travels along the upper exterior of the body to the axillary fold, descends across the back to the axilla, and crosses again to the front of the body.
- This branch continues to ascend along the esophagus, reaching both sides of the base of the tongue and spreading over its lower surface.

---

4. *Cun* is a unit of length equal to ⅓ decimeter.

5. "Red and white" skin refers to the skin that forms the border of the back and palm or sole of the hand or foot.

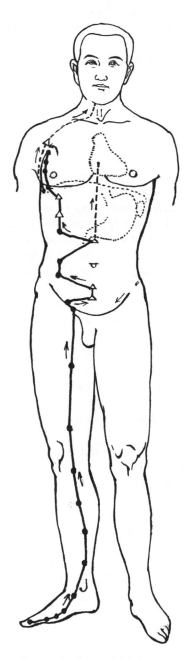

FIGURE 4.5.   Spleen Channel of Foot-Taiyin

- The second branch emerges from the stomach, travels upward through the diaphragm, and disperses into the heart.
- This branch connects with the Heart Channel of Hand-Shaoyin.

THE HEART CHANNEL OF HAND-SHAOYIN (FIGURE 4.6)

- The Heart Channel of Hand-Shaoyin begins in the heart. Emerging, it spreads over the heart system.[6]
- It divides into three branches.
- The first branch passes through the diaphragm to the small intestine.
- The second branch ascends along the side of the esophagus and passes through the pharynx to the "eye system."[7]
- The third branch travels transversely to the lung.
- This branch descends to emerge from the axilla.
- It passes along the back of the medial side of the arm.
- It travels along the inner side of the little finger to its tip.
- It connects with the Small Intestine Channel of Hand-Taiyang at Shaochong point (H 9).

THE SMALL INTESTINE CHANNEL OF HAND-TAIYANG (FIGURE 4.7)

- The Small Intestine Channel of Hand-Taiyang begins from the outside of the tip of the little finger.
- It travels upward along the back of the lateral side of the arm to the shoulder joint.
- It circles around the shoulder and meets the Du Channel at Dazhui point (Du 14).
- It descends into the supraclavicular fossa.
- It divides into two branches.
- The first branch enters the chest, passes through the heart, the diaphragm, the stomach, and finally ends in the small intestine.
- The second branch ascends through the neck up to the cheek, passes the outer canthus and enters the ear.
- This branch travels to the inner canthus along the lower edge of the orbit of the eye.
- It connects with the Urinary Bladder Channel of Foot-Taiyang at Jingming point (UB 1).

6. The "heart system" refers to the tissues connecting the heart with the other *zang-fu* organs.
7. The "eye system" refers to the tissues connecting to the eyeball.

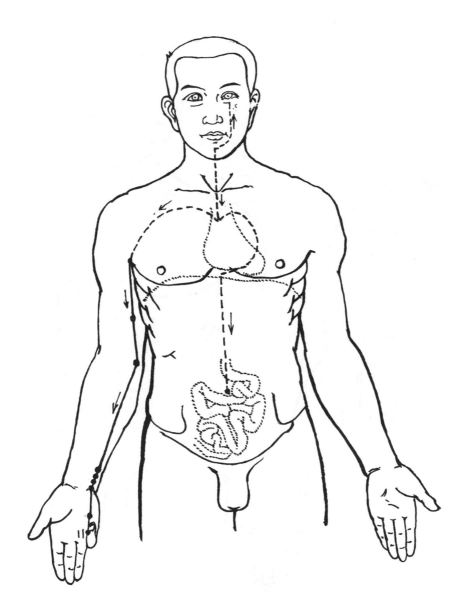

FIGURE 4.6.   Heart Channel of Hand-Shaoyin

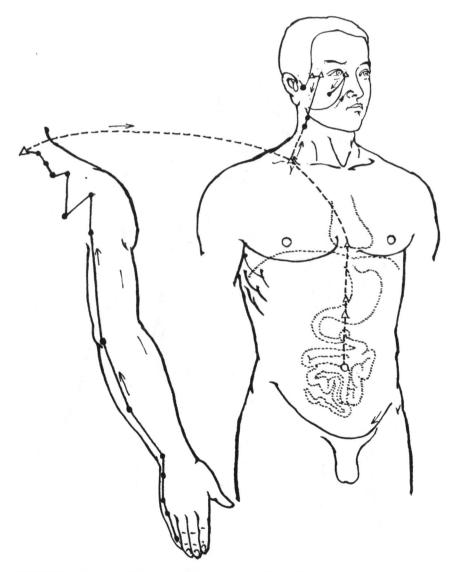

FIGURE 4.7. Small Intestine Channel of Hand-Taiyang

The Urinary Bladder Channel of Foot-Taiyang (Figure 4.8)

- The Urinary Bladder Channel of Foot-Taiyang originates at the inner canthus.
- It ascends to the forehead and spreads over the crown of the head and the upper ear.
- It emerges from the vertex and enters the brain.
- It emerges from the brain, forming branches at the nape of the neck.
- The first branch descends 1.5 *cun* parallel to the vertebral column, to the kidneys and the urinary bladder.
- This branch descends further through the gluteal region, ending in the popliteal fossa.
- The second branch descends from the neck along the medial side of the scapula to the gluteal region, 3 *cun* away from the vertebral column.
- It meets the first branch, descending from the lumbar region in the popliteal fossa.
- It continues down the leg to the lateral side of the tip of the small toe, traveling along the back side of the outer malleolus.
- It connects with the Kidney Channel of Foot-Shaoyin at Zhiyin point (UB 67).

The Kidney Channel of Foot-Shaoyin (Figure 4.9)

- The Kidney Channel of Foot-Shaoyin begins from the underside of the small toe.
- It travels along the sole of the foot to the medial malleolus, where it enters the heel.
- It ascends along the back of the medial side of the tibia to the medial side of the popliteal fossa.
- Ascending up the back of the medial side of the thigh, it travels toward the vertebral column.
- It enters the kidney and urinary bladder.
- Reemerging from the kidney, it ascends straight upward through the liver and diaphragm into the lung.
- It divides into two branches in the lung.
- The first branch ascends along the throat and terminates at both sides of the base of the tongue.
- The second branch enters the heart and travels into the chest.
- It connects with the Pericardium Channel of Hand-Jueyin.

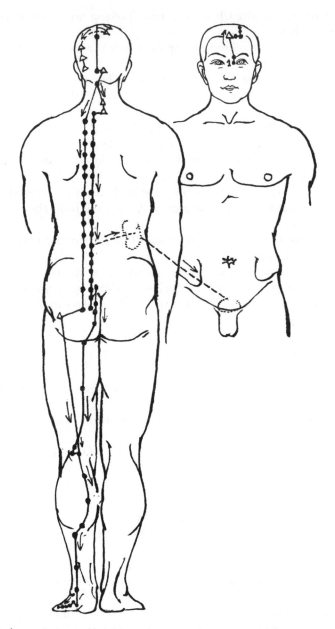

FIGURE 4.8.   Urinary Bladder Channel of Foot-Taiyang

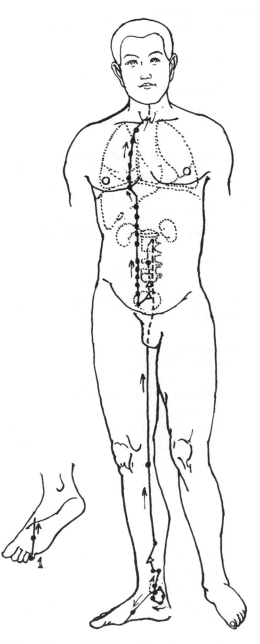

FIGURE 4.9.   Kidney Channel of Foot-Shaoyin

THE PERICARDIUM CHANNEL OF HAND-JUEYIN (FIGURE 4.10)

- The Pericardium Channel of Hand-Jueyin originates in the chest, where it connects with the pericardium, linking the upper, middle, and lower burner.
- A branch arising from the chest travels inside the chest cavity, emerges from the costal region, and ascends to the axilla.
- It travels along the medial side of the arm, terminating at the tip of the middle finger.
- The second branch runs along the ulnar side of the ring finger to its tip.
- It connects with the Triple Burner Channel of Hand-Shaoyang at Guanchong point (SJ 1).

THE TRIPLE BURNER CHANNEL OF HAND-SHAOYANG (FIGURE 4.11)

- The Triple Burner Channel of Hand-Shaoyang originates from the ulnar side of the tip of the ring finger.
- It travels along the dorsal side of the forearm between the radius and ulna.
- It continues along the midline of the lateral side of the extremities, passing the elbow to the shoulder.
- It winds over the shoulder to the supraclavicular fossa.
- In the chest, it divides into two branches at Tanzhong point (Ren 17).
- The first branch travels to the pericardium and then descends through the diaphragm, linking the upper, middle, and lower burners.
- The second branch ascends to the supraclavicular fossa.
- It travels along the surface of the neck, passing the back side of the ear to the upper side.
- It then turns downward to the cheek and terminates in the infraorbital region.
- A subbranch of this second branch originates behind the ear, enters the ear, then reemerges in front of the ear, spreading over the cheek and outer canthus.
- This subbranch connects with the Gallbladder Channel of Foot-Shaoyang at Tongziliao point (GB 1).

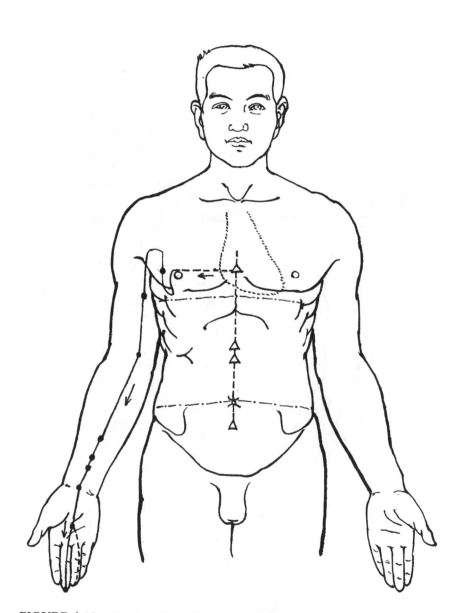

FIGURE 4.10.   Pericardium Channel of Hand-Jueyin

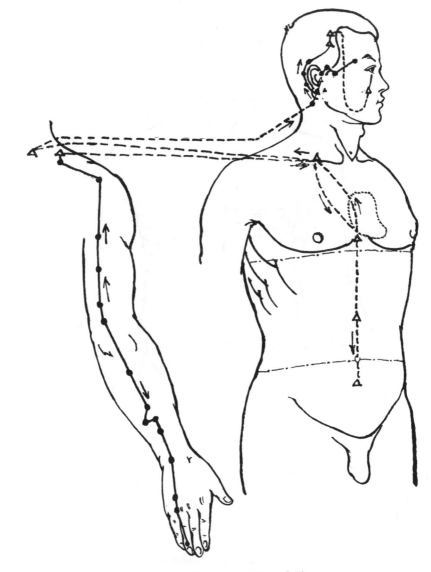

FIGURE 4.11.   Triple Burner Channel of Hand-Shaoyang

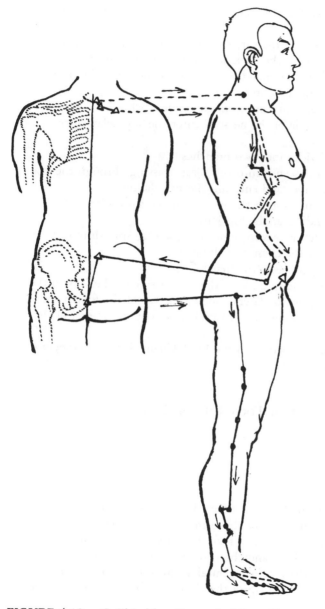
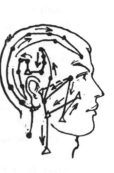

FIGURE 4.12.   Gallbladder Channel of Foot-Shaoyang

The Gallbladder Channel of Foot-Shaoyang (Figure 4.12)

- The Gallbladder Channel of Foot-Shaoyang begins at the outer canthus.
- It curves downward to the region behind the ear, where it divides.
- A small branch enters the ear, reemerges, and passes from the preauricular region to the back side of the outer canthus.
- It then descends to the mandible and on to the infraorbital region, before terminating in the neck.
- The main channel continues from the region behind the ear, along the lateral side of the neck to enter the supraclavicular fossa.
- Here it again divides into two branches.
- The first branch descends into the chest, passing through the diaphragm and the liver and entering the gallbladder.
- It continues down through the groin and the surface area of the pubic region, ending at the hip joint.
- The second branch passes in front of the axilla, spreading over the lateral side of the chest and abdomen.
- At the hip joint, it meets the first branch.
- It descends along the midline of the lateral side of the legs to the malleolus, ending at the lateral side of the tip of the fourth toe.
- A subbranch runs along the dorsum of the foot to the end of the big toe.
- This subbranch connects with the Liver Channel of Foot-Jueyin at Dadun point (Liv 1).

The Liver Channel of Foot-Jueyin (Figure 4.13)

- The Liver Channel of Foot-Jueyin starts from the outside tip of the big toe.
- It passes along the inside of the foot to the front of the medial malleolus.
- It ascends along the front of the medial side of the leg.
- Halfway up the tibia, 8 *cun* above the medial malleolus, it crosses the Spleen Channel of Foot-Taiyin and ascends along the medial side of the knee and thigh to the pubic region.
- It curves around the external genitalia into the lower abdomen.
- It travels upward to the tip of the eleventh rib and then reenters the abdomen.

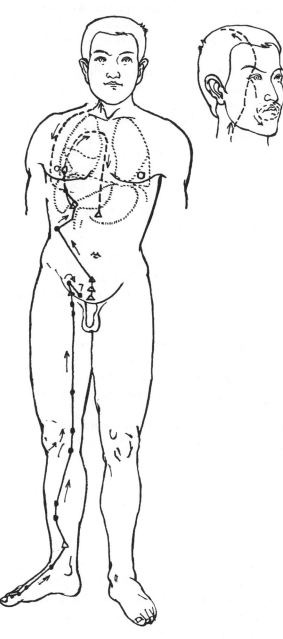

FIGURE 4.13.   Liver Channel of Foot-Jueyin

- It encircles the stomach and enters the liver to communicate with the gallbladder.
- It continues upward, passing through the diaphragm and traversing the costal and upper gastric regions.
- It then enters the lung to meet the Lung Channel of Hand-Tai-yin.
- The channel continues upward through the throat to the nasopharynx and connects with the eyes.
- Here, it divides into two branches.
- The first descends into the cheek and curves around the inner surface of the lips.
- The other emerges at the forehead and continues upward to meet the Du Channel at the vertex.

The Eight Extra Channels

THE DU CHANNEL (FIGURE 4.14) The word *"du"* means to govern." Since the function of the Du Channel is to govern all the *yang* channels of the body, it is thus known as the "confluence of the *yang* channels."

- The Du Channel originates in the uterus or genital organs.
- It descends, emerging at the perineum.
- It then ascends along the midline of the spinal column.
- Passing through the neck, it enters and communicates with the brain.
- From the vertex, it continues down the midline of the forehead to the tip of the nose and then to the upper lip.
- It terminates at the point between the upper lip and the upper gum in the labial frenulum.
- A branch of the Du Channel originates in the sacral bone and passes through the heart, terminating in the kidney.

THE REN CHANNEL (FIGURE 4.15) "Ren" means "responsibility." Since it is responsible for all the *yin* channels, it is known as the "confluence of the *yin* channels." "Ren" also connotes "nourishing." In the woman it is thought to originate in the uterus where the fetus is nourished. Traditional Chinese medicine thus states that "the Ren Channel governs the development of the fetus."

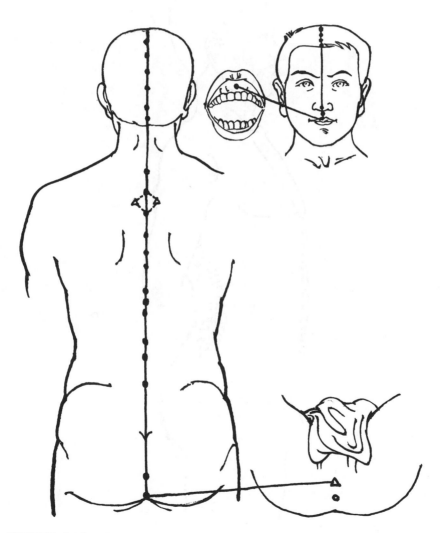

FIGURE 4.14.   Du Channel

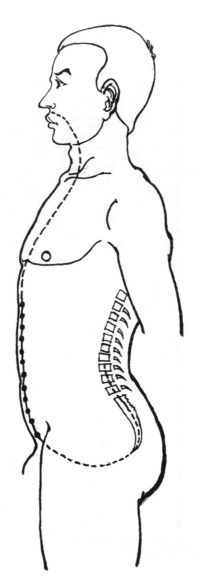

FIGURE 4.15.   Ren Channel

- The Ren Channel originates in the uterus or pelvic cavity.
- It emerges at the perineum and crosses the front of the pubic region in the midline.
- It ascends along the midline through the chest to the inside of the lower lip.
- It then divides into two, encircling the inside of the upper lip.
- The two branches meet at Yinjiao point (Du 28) and go up separately and terminate under the eyes.

THE CHONG CHANNEL (FIGURE 4.16) The Chong Channel is the "confluence of the Twelve Channels." It is also known as the "sea of blood." The Chong Channel controls the *qi* and blood of the entire body, regulating them primarily through the Twelve Principal Channels.

- The Chong Channel originates in the uterus or genital organs.
- It divides into three branches.
- The first branch ascends along the posterior abdominal cavity into the spinal column.
- The second branch ascends along the anterior abdominal cavity, traverses the chest, enters the throat, and encircles the lips.
- The third branch emerges at the perineum, descends along the medial side of the thigh, and terminates between the big toe and the second toe.

THE DAI CHANNEL (FIGURE 4.17) "Dai" means "belt." The Dai Channel is seen as a belt binding the *yin* and *yang* channels. Hence, traditional Chinese medicine states that "all channels are bound by the Dai Channel."

- The Dai Channel starts just below the ribcage.
- It runs transversely around the waist.

THE YINQIAO CHANNEL AND YANGQIAO CHANNEL (FIGURES 4.18, 4.19) *"Qiao"* means "light and nimble." Working as a pair, the Yinqiao and Yangqiao Channels govern much of the motion of the body. The Yangqiao Channel governs the *yang* on both sides of the body while the Yinqiao Channel governs the *yin*. Both channels nourish the eyes, controlling their opening and closing. They also govern the movement of the lower extremities.

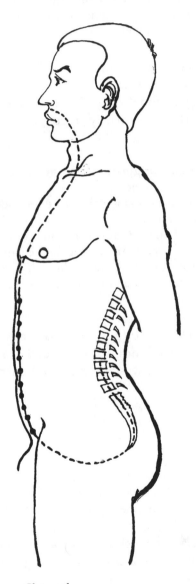

FIGURE 4.16. Chong Channel

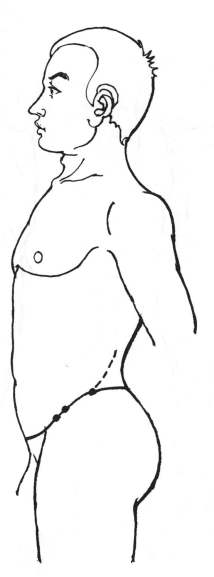

FIGURE 4.17.   Dai Channel

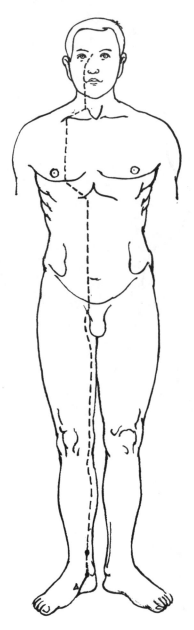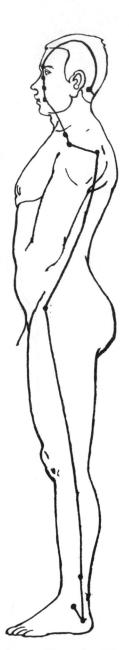

FIGURE 4.18. Yinqiao Channel **FIGURE 4.19. Yangqiao Channel**

- The Yinqiao Channel originates in the heel and ascends along the front of the body.
- It ascends first to the medial malleolus.
- It then travels straight up along the back of the medial side of the leg to the external genitalia.
- Traveling along the surface of the abdomen, it ascends into the supraclavicular fossa.
- It ascends adjacent to the Adam's apple, ending in the inner canthus, where it communicates with the Yangqiao Channel.
- The Yangqiao Channel originates at the heel and travels upward along the back of the body.
- It ascends along the external malleolus and up the lateral side of the leg.
- It passes through the waist to travel along the back of the ribcage.
- It ascends to the shoulder and the supraclavicular fossa, then travels up the neck to the corner of the mouth.
- At the inner canthus it communicates with the Yinqiao Channel.
- It continues to the forehead, following the Urinary Bladder of Foot-Taiyang.
- It terminates at the nape of the neck, where it meets the Gallbladder Channel of Foot-Shaoyang.

THE YINWEI CHANNEL AND THE YANGWEI CHANNEL (FIGURES 4.20, 4.21) *"Wei"* means "link." The Yinwei Channel links the three *yin* channels; it is thus known as "the regulating channel of *yin*." Similarly, the Yangwei Channel links the three *yang* channels and is known as "the regulating channel of *yang*."

- The Yinwei Channel originates at the medial side of the tibia where the three *yin* channels meet.
- It ascends along the medial side of the leg to the abdomen, where it communicates with the Spleen Channel of Foot-Taiyin.
- It continues to ascend to the ribcage, where it joins the Liver Channel of Foot-Jueyin.
- It terminates in the pharynx, where it communicates with the Ren Channel.
- The Yangwei Channel originates in the external malleolus.
- Running parallel to the Gallbladder Channel of Foot-Shaoyang, it ascends along the lateral side of the trunk and the back of the axillary fold to the shoulder.

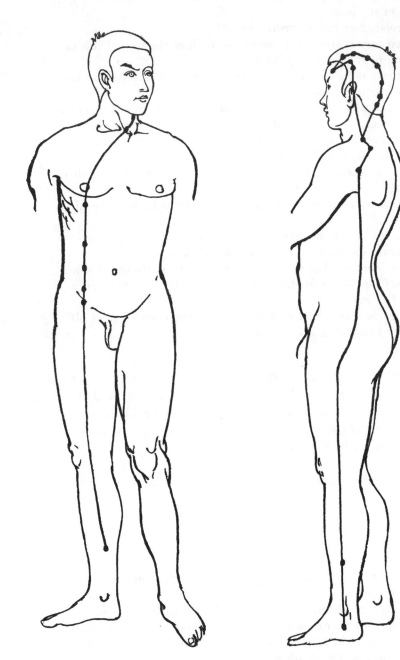

FIGURE 4.20.   Yinwei Channel   FIGURE 4.21.   Yangwei Channel

- It travels to the forehead via the neck.
- It then returns to the nape where it terminates by meeting the Du Channel.

THE PATHWAY OF DISEASE

The interstitial space between the skin and flesh opens when pathogenic factors invade. Consequently they succeed in entering the collaterals, channels, and viscera, step by step.

"Treatise on the Correspondence of the Skin
to the Channels" in *Plain Questions*

Since the channels are the paths through which *qi* and blood circulate, they are also the paths for transmission of exogenous pathogenic factors from the skin to the space between the flesh and skin, and ultimately to the internal organs. The sequence of transmission of pathogenic factors—that is, from the skin to the Tendon/Muscle Channels to the Divergent Channels to the Twelve Principal Channels to the *fu* organs and finally to the *zang* organs—corresponds to the layers of concentric cylinders described earlier.

The body's first line of defense is in the outer cylinder, where the *wei qi,* or defensive *qi,* guards against the invasion of pathogenic factors. If the *wei qi* is insufficient, the pathogenic factors may launch an attack along the channels at points where there is functional failure—a block or stagnation, for example. Typically, this attack proceeds from the superficial to the interior parts of the body.

However, the transmission of exogenous pathogenic factors does not always follow this pattern. In some cases, the *zang-fu* organs are affected immediately. The factors that determine the path of transmission are: (1) how well the channels are functioning; (2) how well the *zang-fu* organs are functioning; and (3) the relative strength of the pathogenic factors versus the overall level of resistance of the body.

In addition to exogenous pathogenic factors, illness may originate in the channel system itself. A functional weakness or failure of a channel will lead to a weakening of channel *qi.* Such disturbances of channel *qi* will first affect the circulating and nourishing abilities of the channel system.

Since the channels in a healthy body regulate the relationship between the *zang* and *fu* organs, they will also transmit disease among these organs in an unhealthy body. As was explained in the previous chapter, liver trouble may affect the spleen; heart trouble that results from the retention of water due to a deficiency of kidney *qi* may affect the lungs; and pathogenic heat from the heart may be transmitted to the small intestine. The channel system provides the functional link between the organs—the link that leads to these and other pathological relationships.

Finally, the pathological pathway works in reverse. A disease that begins in an internal organ will eventually lead to a disturbance on the exterior of the body. Furthermore, the location of the disturbance is generally predictable. Thus, the ancient Chinese noted that:

> The invasion of the lung and heart by pathogenic factors causes the stagnation of *qi* in both elbows. If the liver is attacked, the stagnation of *qi* occurs in the armpit. When the spleen and kidney are affected, *qi* collects in the groin and in the knee, respectively.
> "Treatise on Exogenous Pathogenic Factors
> and Treatment" in *Miraculous Pivot*

The elbows, armpits, groin, and the backs of the knees are regions where the channels and collaterals pass in their course of circulation. The stagnation of *qi* at one of these points leads to an obstruction in the flow of *qi* and blood, which often results in pain. Common pains connected with disease in the internal organs are: aching in the chest and soreness of the arms in cases of lung disease; aching in the chest and trembling of the hands in cases of heart disease; distending pain in the costal region as a result of liver trouble; abdominal pain and soreness in the groin in spleen disease; pain in the lumbar region and weakness in the knees in kidney disorders; swollen gums and toothaches due to the accumulation of heat in the large intestine; and earache and deafness in the so-called upward rush or flaring of gallbladder fire.

Because of the links provided by the channels between the surface of the body and the interior organs, these exterior pains can be used diagnostically. However, they must be evaluated cautiously. A disturbance may begin on the body's exterior and never reach an internal organ; thus, an external pain does not necessarily indicate a disease in the corresponding organ. Similarly, a disease beginning in one of the *zang-fu* organs may not immediately produce an external manifestation. For example, in the case of strokes, the early stages show no obvious signs on the exterior of the body. Later, however, even if the internal situation is alleviated, there are external aftereffects, such as paralysis, that remain in the extremities. This pattern can be attributed to the eventual disturbance of the circulating function in the extremities and hence the disturbance of channel *qi*.

USING THE CHANNELS TO DIAGNOSE
AND TREAT DISEASE

Knowing the effects of the Twelve Principal Channels in the physiology and pathology of the body, one may ascertain the origin of disease. Knowing the functional conditions of the channels, one may understand whether the disease sites are in the upper or lower portions of the body.

"Treatise on Defensive *Qi*" in *Miraculous Pivot*

By observing tender spots and the color of the face, as well as the upper, lower, left, and right portions of the body, one may ascertain the symptom-complexes of the channels and their cold or warm nature.

"Treatise on Functions" in *Miraculous Pivot*

As indicated above, the channel system can be used, with caution, to diagnose disease since it systematically reflects the pathological symptoms of the internal organs—both in the channels themselves and on the body surface. The location and type of external symptoms, together with their order of occurrence, indicates which channel and which *zang-fu* organ is affected. In fact, "Treatise on Functions" quoted above, develops a system for differentiating symptom-complexes based on the theory of the channels.

The channel theory also provides an extensive foundation for the treatment of disease. It is at the heart of many traditional therapies, including acupuncture, therapeutic massage, and the use of herbal medicines. The treatment points for acupuncture and massage, for example, are determined by the theory of the channel systems. So is the more recent practice of acupuncture anesthesia. If a channel is obstructed, the practitioner may choose points on a neighboring channel or distant points on the obstructed channel to administer acupuncture or massage. Through this process, the practitioner can intervene in the regulation of blood and *qi* to effect a cure.

TABLE 4.2.   Symptoms of the Twelve Principal Channels

Each channel has associated with it a set of symptoms that appear when it is not functioning properly. This chart is a summary of some of the major symptoms associated with the Twelve Principal Channels. It is not comprehensive, however. For a more complete understanding, see chapter 8, on diagnosis.

The Lung Channel of Hand-Taiyin
    Fullness in the chest
    Pain in the supraclavicular fossa
    Cough
    Dyspnea
    Asthma
    Aching along the anterior border of the medial side of upper extremities
    Pain in the shoulder and back
    Sore throat

The Large Intestine Channel of Hand-Yangming
    Aching of the lower teeth
    Sore throat
    Epistaxis
    Serous nasal discharge
    Thirst
    Swollen neck
    Aching and impaired motion along the anterior border of the lateral side of the upper extremities and shoulders

The Stomach Channel of Foot-Yangming
    High fever and perspiration
    Epistaxis
    Lip rash
    Facial paralysis
    Headache
    Sore throat
    Swollen neck
    Mania
    Abdominal distension
    Borborygmus
    Edema
    Pain and impaired motion along the anterolateral side of the lower extremities, the dorsum of the foot, and the middle toe

The Spleen Channel of the Foot-Taiyin
    Rigidity of the tongue
    Vomiting
    Sluggishness
    Abdominal distension and pain
    Pain or cold sensation in the medial side of the lower extremities

Impaired motion of the big toe
Jaundice

The Heart Channel of Hand-Shaoyin
Pain in the cardiac or hypochondriac region
Thirst
Aching or cold sensation along the posterior border of the medial side of the
upper extremities
Elevated temperature in the palms

The Small Intestine Channel of Hand-Taiyang
Deafness
Jaundice
Sore throat
Swelling and pain in the mandible and neck, causing stiff neck
Aching in the shoulder, arm, and posterior border of the medial side of the
upper extremities

The Urinary Bladder Channel of Foot-Taiyang
Stiff neck or headache
Pain or impairment of motion in the lumbar region
Swelling and pain in the eyeball
Epistaxis
Hemiplegia
Pain or impairment of motion along the course of the channel
Ophthalmological disorders
Hemorrhoids
Malaria
Mania
Scabies

The Kidney Channel of Foot-Shaoyin
Dyspnea
Hemoptysis
Dizziness
Dryness of the tongue
Dryness and swelling of the pharynx
Diarrhea
Lumbago
Muscular atrophy and cold sensation in the lower extremities
Elevated temperature in the sole of the foot

The Pericardium Channel of Hand-Jueyin
Palpitations
Restlessness
Fullness in the chest and hypochondriac region
Angina pectoris
Mania

TABLE 4.2.   Symptoms of the Twelve Principal Channels (Continued)

Spasms of the upper extremities
Elevated temperature in the palm
Swelling of the axilla

The Triple Burner Channel of Hand-Shaoyang
Deafness
Sore throat
Pain in the retroauricular region, shoulder and forearm
Impaired motion of the little finger or index finger

The Gallbladder Channel of Foot-Shaoyang
Alternating spells of fever and chills
Bitter taste in the mouth
Frequent sighing
Pain in the hypochondriac region
Migraine
Tuberculous cervical lymphadenitis
Malaria
Pain or impaired motion in the thigh, the knee, the lateral side of the tibia,
   and the fourth toe

The Liver Channel of Foot-Jueyin
Stiffness and pain in the hypochondriac region
Fullness in the chest
Vomiting
Diarrhea
Hernia
Retention of urine
Lumbago
Abdominal pain in women

The transmitting function of the channels also determines the action of a drug on the diseased part of the body. Part of the historical tradition of Chinese herbal medicine is a theory that describes the "medicines finding their way to the channels."[8] According to this theory, certain drugs in certain quantities are beneficial to the channels of certain organs. The effect of any given drug depends on its flavor, property, and type of action. For example, *Herba Ephedra,* which has a pungent taste and warm properties, can enter the Lung and Urinary Bladder Channels. *Radix Puerariae,* with a pungent but sweet flavor and moderate properties, can enter the Spleen and Stom-

8. These principles of drug actions and their relationship to the channels are described in volume 2, chapter 2.

TABLE 4.3. Symptoms of the Eight Extra Channels

The Du Channel
Stiffness and pain in the spinal column
Opisthotonos
Mental disorders
Infantile convulsions

The Ren Channel
Hernia
Leukorrhea
Mass in the lower abdomen
Menstrual irregularities
Miscarriage
Sterility

The Chong Channel
Menstrual irregularities
Amenorrhea
Uterine bleeding
Deficient lactation
Hematemesis

The Dai Channel
Leukorrhea
Prolapse of the uterus
Fullness of the abdomen
Weakness of the lumbar region

The Yinqiao Channel
Inversion of the foot
Sore throat
Hypersomnia

The Yangqiao Channel
Eversion of the foot
Mania
Insomia
Pain and redness of the inner canthus

The Yinwei Channel
Pain in the chest, heart, and stomach

The Yangwei Channel
Recurrences of chills and fever

ach Channels. *Radix Bupleurum Chinese,* with a bitter taste and moderate properties, can enter the Liver and Gallbladder channels. *Rhizoma Gastrodia Elata* has a sweet taste and warm properties and can therefore enter the Liver Channel.

Knowing the function of the channels, the practitioner can thus predict that these herbal medicines will have the following effects: *Herba Ephedra Sinica* is beneficial in dispersing lung *qi* and relieving cough and asthma. It is also a good diuretic. *Radix Puerariae* can be used to alleviate excessive stomach heat, thirst, or diarrhea due to deficiency in the spleen since it promotes the production of body fluid and the ascending activity of *yang qi*. *Radix Bupleurum Chinese* can alleviate stagnation of liver *qi* and hypochondriac pain because it can relieve stagnancy of *qi* in the liver. *Rhizoma Gastrodia Elata* is beneficial in subduing hyperfunction of the liver and endogenous wind; in addition, it is used to treat vertigo due to excess liver *yang*.

Drugs can also serve as conductors for other drugs that do not readily enter the target channel. In this way, they can direct the work of these latter drugs to achieve curative effects that they themselves cannot produce.

IN SUMMARY

The channel system has three functions in the body: (1) communication among related parts of the body; (2) regulation of the activities of the *zang-fu* organs; and (3) distribution of *qi* and the other basic life materials throughout the body.

The channel system consists of several different types of pathways. The Twelve Principal Channels connect the internal organs to the surface of the body; each corresponds to either a *zang* or a *fu* organ. The Eight Extra Channels help assure the steady flow of blood and *qi*. The Divergent Channels also link the body surface to the internal organs, but in general they follow a more superficial course than the Twelve Principal Channels. The Connecting Channels maintain communication among the Principal Channels. The Tendon/Muscle Channels carry the flow of *qi* along the surface of the body. The Cutaneous Regions of the Twelve Principal Channels reflect the condition of the channels and internal organs. The Superficial and Tertiary Channels support the activities of the other channels in distributing blood and *qi* throughout the body.

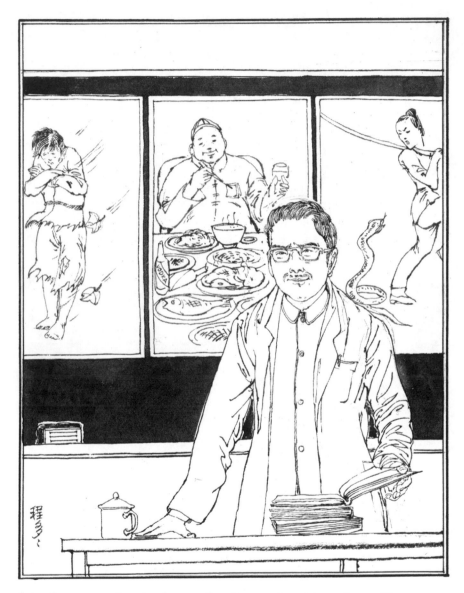

A teacher presenting the theory of pathogenesis to his students. The posters in the background illustrate three factors causing disease.

———— ◆ ————

CHAPTER FIVE

Etiology:
The Cause of Disease

Thousands of illnesses are no more than three kinds of injury.
Synopsis of the Golden Chamber

ETIOLOGY IS THE study of the cause of disease. In traditional Chinese medicine, disease is classified according to symptom-complexes. The study of etiology in Chinese medicine is thus a study of the factors that produce symptom-complexes.

The Chinese concept of etiology has its origins in the *Classic of Internal Medicine,* which identified two causes of disease: climatic factors and dysfunction of the human body. These causes were labeled *yang* and *yin,* respectively:

> Pathogenic agents may come from the interior of the body, which pertains to *yin,* or from the exterior environment, which pertains to *yang.* What comes from *yang* is the result of abnormal climatic factors, including wind, rain, cold, or summer heat. What comes from *yin* may result from improper diet, irregular life, intemperate sexuality, extreme joy or anger.
>
> "Treatise on the Regulation of Channels,"
> in *Plain Questions*

The Synopsis of the Golden Chamber, written in the third century, expanded these two causes of disease to three "injuries." First was injury of the channels and collaterals by pathogenic factors that could then invade the internal organs. Second was injury to the body surface by pathogenic factors that could then invade the four extremities, the nine body orifices, and the vessels, eventually obstructing the flow of blood. The third type of injury was a mixed category that included such causes as intemperate sexuality, wounds, and animal or insect bites.

These three categories of injury developed into "the theory of three causes of disease." They have come to be known as "endogenous" pathogenic factors, "exogenous" pathogenic factors, and pathogenic factors that are "neither endogenous nor exogenous." Etiology in traditional Chinese medicine is the study of these pathogenic factors, of their relationship with each other, and their influence on the functioning of the body.

PATHOGENIC FACTORS: THE CONCEPT OF "EVIL"

The pathogenic factors of traditional Chinese medicine are not the pathogens of Western medicine.[1] In Chinese medicine, pathogenic factors are harmful influences that disturb the relative internal balance of the human body or the balance between the body and the external environment. The literal translation of "pathogenic factor" in Chinese is simply *"evil qi."*

Any pathogenic factor can cause disease only when it disrupts the "unity of opposites" in the body—when it results in a disturbance of the balance between *yin* and *yang* and between *qi* and blood in the organs and tissues. An attack on the body by an exogenous pathogenic factor is only the external cause. It is the *condition* under which disease can occur. But the existence of the condition does not mean that the disease must necessarily occur. The occurrence and development of disease depends on internal (or endogenous) factors: the mental state, the functional condition of the internal organs, and the body's defensive strength and regenerative ability.

When the balance of the body is disturbed by different combinations of exogenous and endogenous pathogenic factors, different symptom-complexes appear. The principal task of the clinician is to

1. The Chinese concept of pathogenic factors has traditionally included the idea of the "epidemic pathogenic agent" as one type of pathogenic factor. The microbes and bacteria of modern science have thus been easily incorporated into this concept. However, they remain a very small part of the general class of pathogenic factors.

"trace the causes of a disease by differentiating symptom-complexes."[2] The principal task of the student of etiology is to describe the process by which various pathogenic factors interact to produce distinct symptom-complexes.

THE SIX EXCESSES: CLIMATIC FACTORS

The ancient Chinese categorized the principal exogenous pathogenic factors according to climatic characteristics: wind, cold, heat, dampness, dryness, and fire. These climatic factors correspond to normal seasonal changes and, under normal conditions, are known as the "six *qi*." The growth and development of living things depend on the existence of these six *qi* and man has adapted to them to a certain extent. Thus, the normal six *qi* will not attack the body and cause disease.

If the six *qi* become abnormal or excessive as in cases of abrupt and extreme changes in environmental conditions, or if the body's resistance is too weak to adapt to these variations, the six *qi* can become the "six excesses"—pathogenic factors that destroy the physiological equilibrium of the human body, thus causing disease.

The six exogenous pathogenic factors are often related to seasonal changes in weather. However, they should not be interpreted strictly as climatic factors. They represent a system for categorizing pathogenic factors that have a particular effect on the body. Accordingly, they may include such environmental factors as toxic chemicals or microorganisms, provided these have the same effect on the body as one of the six climatic factors.

Typically, disease is not the result of a single climatic factor. One or more factors may invade the body to cause disease. Also, in the course of a disease, various of the six excesses may interact, influencing one another, or one may be transformed into the other, leading to corresponding changes in the nature of the disease.

2. For example, if a patient is suffering from loss of appetite, abdominal distension, loose stools, and general sluggishness, and if he or she has a thick tongue coating, the Chinese practitioner would assert that the cause of the disease is "pathogenic dampness," explaining that pathogenic dampness has invaded the spleen and impaired its normal functions of transporting and transforming. The remedy would be an invigoration of the spleen to dispel dampness. In this case, "pathogenic dampness" is the cause of the symptom-complex that explains all of the symptoms presented.

Exogenous pathogenic factors invade the body from the exterior via the body surface, the mouth, and/or the nose. They eventually affect specific internal organs; this "corresponding" relationship between the organs and the six climatic factors means that certain diseases are more likely to occur in one season than another.

While the six excesses are generally exogenous pathogenic factors, wind, cold, heat, dampness, dryness, and fire may also appear as endogenous factors. These originate in the interior of the body due to a dysfunction of the internal organs rather than invading the body from outside. However, their nature and pathological effects are often similar to those of the six exogenous excesses. These pathological effects may be summarized as follows:

Wind

In the traditional Chinese view of the world, wind is said to prevail in spring. But pathogenic wind, and the diseases that it causes, are not confined to spring. They can occur in any season. Such diseases, by analogy to the wind, have the following characteristics:

WIND DISEASES AFFECT THE *YANG* PARTS OF THE BODY.

Wind is a *yang* pathogenic factor. It is a shapeless air current, coming and going rapidly. It rises one moment and subsides the next. It is changeable and all pervasive. Its movement is outward and upward. Pathogenic wind thus tends to attack the *yang* parts of the body: the body surface and the upper body. Symptoms usually appear in the head, body surface, and limbs. Since pathogenic wind attacks the body surface, it may cause the pores to open. Sweating and aversion to wind will then appear as symptoms.

WIND DISEASES BEGIN ABRUPTLY, AND THEIR SYMPTOMS MIGRATE TO DIFFERENT POSITIONS IN THE BODY.

Wind, especially pathogenic wind, occurs in gusts and is characterized by rapid change. Similarly, diseases caused by pathogenic wind begin abruptly. Their symptoms are variable, migrating to different positions of the body. Rheumatism is an example of a disease caused predominantly by pathogenic wind (although cold and dampness are also factors). It is marked by migratory pain in the joints and is often called "wind arthritis" in Chinese. Other examples of disease caused by pathogenic wind—and therefore with migratory characteristics—are allergic rashes, urticaria, strokes, hemiplegia, distortion of the face (Bell's palsy), and facial paralysis.

WIND DISEASES ARE ACCOMPANIED BY ABNORMAL MOVEMENT.

Wind is characterized by constant movement. It is said that the wind proves its existence by causing the branches and leaves of the trees to sway and rock. Diseases caused by pathogenic wind usually lead to abnormal motion, with symptoms such as dizziness, tremors, convulsions, rigidity of the neck, and opisthotonos (spasm in which the spine and extremities are bent with convexity forward). This movement is said to be due to the pathological changes of wind stirring.

WIND DISEASES USUALLY RESULT FROM A COMBINATION OF PATHOGENIC FACTORS.

The liver is the organ primarily affected by pathogenic wind. Exogenous pathogenic wind may enter the body and eventually invade the liver, disrupting its function. At the same time, internal disturbances of the liver—liver *qi* is susceptible to abnormal stirring, and liver *yang* is likely to be preponderant—are the source of endogenous pathogenic wind.

Table 5.1 describes the symptom complexes that commonly result from pathogenic wind.

TABLE 5.1. Symptom-Complexes of Pathogenic Wind

Exogenous Wind

This is the common cold. The body surface is attacked by pathogenic wind, leading to fever, aversion to wind, sweating, scratchy throat, cough, nasal congestion, and watery snivel. The pulse is slow and floating.

Wind-Cold

Pathogenic wind associated with cold leads to an intolerance of wind and cold, fever, headache or general aching, congested nose and watery snivel, and a loud cough. It is marked by the absence of sweating (hypohidrosis). The pulse is floating and tight.

TABLE 5.1.   Symptom-Complexes of Pathogenic Wind (Continued)

Wind-Heat

Pathogenic wind complicated by heat leads to symptoms of fever without aversion to cold (or with slight aversion to wind), perspiration, distending pain in the head, swollen and sore throat, reddened eyes with distension and pain, photophobia, thirst and dryness of the throat, cough, shortness of breath, thick yellow sputum, constipation, dark yellow urine, and a thin yellow coating on the tongue. If wind-heat attacks the vessels of the lung (and the stomach, in some cases), bleeding may occur, with hemoptysis, epistaxis, and hematemesis. The pulse is floating and rapid.

Wind-Warmth

Typical of the early stages of many infectious diseases, this symptom-complex includes high fever, headache, aversion to wind, and sweating. If the pathogenic factor transforms into heat after penetrating the interior of the body, symptoms will include a burning sensation in the body, profuse sweating, cough, feeling of suffocation in the chest, delirium, and a dark red tongue without coating. The pulse is floating and rapid.

Wind-Dampness

Two conditions commonly result from this combination of pathogenic factors: (1) attack by wind associated with dampness producing, in addition to symptoms of the common cold, pain in the limbs, general sluggishness, a sensation of distension in the head, loss of appetite, nausea, scanty urine, and loose stools; and (2) arthritis caused by wind-dampness, marked by migrating pain in the joints and muscles, with pain corresponding to changes in the weather.

Endogenous Wind

Endogenous stirring of wind in the liver produces symptoms of dizziness, spasm in the limbs, convulsions, numbness, rigidity and sudden coma, facial paralysis, and hemiplegia. These occur as a result of abnormalities in the sinews, eyes, and mental activities, which, in turn, result from the transformation of liver *yang* into pathogenic wind. These abnormalities may also be caused by a deficiency of blood or by extreme heat.

Cold

Cold is the prevailing climatic condition in winter. Therefore, the natural phenomena that occur in this season—such as freezing and coagulation—illustrate the characteristics of diseases caused by pathogenic cold. These characteristics may be defined as follows:

COLD DISEASES INHIBIT THE BODY'S *YANG QI.*

Cold is a *yin* pathogenic factor. Pathogenic cold therefore tends to suppress the defensive *yang* of the body by blocking its dispersion on the surface of the body. The result is the symptom-complex of exogenous cold. (See table 5.2.) If pathogenic cold invades the interior of the body, the *yang* functioning of the spleen and stomach is impaired, leading to a dysfunction in the transport and distribution of nutrients and water.

COLD DISEASES ARE ACCOMPANIED BY PAIN.

The continuous smooth flow of *qi,* blood, and body fluid throughout the body depends on the warming, impelling influence of *yang qi.* Since pathogenic cold impairs *yang qi,* it produces stagnation: the circulation of blood and *qi* is retarded. This stagnation causes pain. Typically, an attack of pathogenic cold on the body surface will produce headache and general aching. If it obstructs the flow of *qi* in the internal organs, pathogenic cold will lead to pain in the abdomen.

COLD DISEASES ARE CHARACTERIZED BY CONTRACTION.

Cold produces contraction, and pathogenic cold tends to cause contraction of the vessels in particular. If it attacks the body surface, the pores of the skin, the muscular vessels, and the interstitial spaces of the muscles will close tightly, hindering the dispersal of *yang qi:* If the channels and vessels contract and obstruct the circulation of *qi* and blood, muscular contractions, spasms, and rigidity of the limbs will appear. Spasmodic pain in the testes and lower abdomen, in particular, indicates contraction of the Liver Channel by pathogenic cold.

COLD DISEASES AFFECT THE KIDNEY.

The kidney is the organ most closely associated with pathogenic cold. Exogenous pathogenic cold and dampness will usually elicit pathological changes in the kidney, leading to low back pain, for

TABLE 5.2.   Symptom-Complexes of Pathogenic Cold

Superficial Exogenous Cold

Superficial invasion of pathogenic cold produces intolerance of cold, fever without sweating, rigidity and pains in the neck, aching in the joints, cough, and asthmatic breathing. The pulse is floating and tight.

Interior Exogenous Cold

Penetration of the interior by exogenous cold injures the stomach and spleen or impairs the *yang* of the spleen and kidney. Symptoms are aversion to cold; shivering, numbness, and coldness in the limbs; livid face and purple lips; diarrhea, intestinal rumbling; abdominal pain that can be relieved by heat; loss of appetite; vomiting; spasms of the jaw muscles; aphasia; contractures or rigidity of the limbs; contracted tongue; and retracted testicles. The pulse is deep, slow, and thready.

Wind-Cold-Dampness, with Predominant Cold

If pathogenic wind, cold, and dampness linger in the channels, collaterals, and joints and if cold is the prevalent pathogenic factor, the result will be arthralgia or arthritis with severe joint pains. This pain is relieved by heat and aggravated by cold. The pulse is taut and tight.

Endogenous Cold

This symptom-complex is a state of functional decline due to general deficiency of *yang* and *qi*. Major symptoms are intolerance of cold and preference for warmth, cool limbs, cold hands and feet, vomiting of clear fluid, diarrhea with watery stools containing undigested food, profuse clear urine, lassitude and sleepiness, localized cold and pain. The pulse is deep and slow.

example. At the same time, insufficiency of kidney *yang* is the source of endogenous or internal pathogenic cold.

The symptom complexes of pathogenic cold appear in table 5.2.

Heat

Unlike other pathogenic factors, pathogenic heat results directly from climatic conditions. It appears only in hot, summerlike conditions and is therefore also known as pathogenic summer-heat. Because it is directly related to environmental conditions, pathogenic summer-heat is always an exogenous pathogenic factor.

Diseases of pathogenic heat have the following characteristics:

DISEASES OF SUMMER-HEAT LEAD TO AN EXUBERANCE OF *YANG QI*.

Summer-heat is a *yang* pathogenic factor and is liable to attack the secondary defensive system of the body. It produces an exuberance of *yang qi,* which, in turn, produces high fever, thirst, perspiration, and an overflowing pulse.

SUMMER-HEAT DISEASES DISPLAY A DECREASE IN BODY FLUID.

A characteristic quality of summer-heat is its dissipating action. In the human body, this action leads to a consumption of fluids and *qi.* Heat causes the muscles, tissues, and interstitial spaces of the body to open. Excessive sweating results. Profuse sweating means that body fluid is consumed faster than it can be replaced. At the same time, original *qi* is reduced since *qi* may escape after a great loss of body fluid. This deficiency of *qi* leads to hypofunctioning of the body.

TABLE 5.3.   Symptom-Complexes of Pathogenic Heat

Exposure to Summer-Heat

A mild form of disease, this symptom-complex includes a sensation of fever, perspiration, dizziness, headache, thirst with desire to drink fluids, dry lips, general lassitude, nausea, and a thick, white coating of the tongue. The pulse is slippery and rapid.

Heat-Stroke

A more severe form of exposure to summer-heat (or sometimes the result of a very high fever), this symptom-complex is characterized by giddiness, nausea, a feeling of suffocation in the chest, feverishness, profuse sweating, shortness of breath, and restlessness. In the most severe cases, there may be a coma with asthmatic breathing and coldness of limbs. The pulse is overflowing.

Damp-Heat

Pathogenic heat combines with dampness to produce alternating spells of chills and fever, restlessness, thirst, or thirst with no desire to drink fluids, a feeling of suffocation in the chest, nausea, poor appetite, general lassitude and sluggishness, loose stools, reduced urination, and a thick white or yellow coating of the tongue. The pulse is feeble and rapid.

DISEASES OF PATHOGENIC HEAT OFTEN OCCUR IN COMBINATION WITH PATHOGENIC DAMPNESS.

Summer is often a season of dampness as well as heat. The evaporation of liquids that is fostered by heat increases the humidity in the air. This climatic condition can lead to the symptom-complex of heat-dampness. This and other symptom-complexes of pathogenic summer-heat are summarized in table 5.3.

Dampness

In traditional Chinese thought, dampness is the prevailing climate factor of late summer, which, in China, is the time of highest humidity. Diseases of pathogenic dampness, however, can occur any time the weather has been wet and rainy for several days. They may also attack a person who has been dwelling in a damp place, working on the water, or wearing clothing wet from rain, water, or sweat. Like the other excesses, pathogenic dampness may originate in the interior of the body as well. In this case, a dysfunction of the spleen leads to water retention.

Diseases of pathogenic dampness have the following characteristic features:

DISEASES OF DAMPNESS IMPAIR *YANG QI.*

Dampness is a *yin* pathogenic factor and is therefore apt to disturb the normal flow of *qi;* especially it impairs *yang qi.* In the case of pathogenic dampness, it is primarily spleen *yang* that is impaired. The transport and distribution of nutrients and water become abnormal, and water is retained by the body. Symptoms such as diarrhea, scanty urine, edema, and ascites appear. In general, pathogenic dampness attacks the *yin* parts of the body.

DISEASES OF PATHOGENIC DAMPNESS ARE CHARACTERIZED BY HEAVINESS AND TURBIDITY.

Dampness in nature is weighty and turbid; it is characterized by downward motion. In the body, pathogenic dampness produces feelings of sluggishness. The head often feels as though it is tightly bandaged. Edema appears, especially in the legs. Pathogenic dampness also tends to produce turbid excretions from the body: gum in the eyes, sticky loose stools, turbid urine, massive, foul-smelling vaginal discharge, oozing eczema (sometimes with a yellowish discharge), or even ulcers.

DISEASES OF PATHOGENIC DAMPNESS TEND TO LINGER AND ARE DIFFICULT TO CURE.

Among the natural characteristics of dampness are viscosity, stagnation, and diffusion. These characteristics lead to diseases that are often lingering. Relapses are frequent. Also, illnesses resulting from pathogenic dampness tend to spread over the body, rather than confining themselves to a single, localized area. Stagnation appears in the large intestine as tenesmus—the sensation of needing to defecate. Accumulation of dampness also produces excess phlegm, leading to symptoms of profuse sputum, nausea, vomiting, and an oppressive

TABLE 5.4. Symptom-Complexes of Pathogenic Dampness

Exogenous Dampness

Dampness which interferes with the normal flow of *qi* produces a feeling of oppression in the chest and upper abdomen, vomiting and nausea, anorexia, scanty urine, difficulty in urination, and constipation. The pulse is soft, weak and floating.

It may also produce arthralgia or arthritis with fixed pain and heaviness in the joints, impaired motion of the limbs, and/or numbness of the muscles and skin. The pulse is then stringy, weak and floating.

Wind-Dampness, with Predominant Dampness

This symptom-complex is marked by fever that is especially pronounced in the afternoon; fever that is low and not relieved by perspiration; heaviness in the head; general sluggishness; and soreness or pain in the limbs. The pulse is rapid, weak and floating.

Endogenous Dampness

This symptom-complex is due to retention of fluids that fail to be transported properly because the spleen is deficient. Symptoms are a poor appetite, stickiness in the mouth, absence of thirst, oppressive feeling in the chest, nausea, feeling of fullness in the abdomen and head, general sluggishness, loose stools, diarrhea, sallow complexion, edema, turbid urine, and—in women—abnormal vaginal discharge. The pulse is thready, weak and floating.

sensation in the chest. Stagnation in the joints leads to arthralgia. In general, such diseases are difficult to cure.

DISEASES OF DAMPNESS ATTACK THE SPLEEN.

When exogenous pathogenic dampness invades the body, it is most likely to affect spleen *yang,* disrupting its transport and distribution. The reverse is also true: when the spleen's functions of transport and distribution are disrupted owing to deficiency, exogenous pathogenic dampness is likely to appear. Endogenous and exogenous dampness often promote each other. Exogenous dampness is more likely to attack the body if the metabolism of water is already impaired due to deficiency of spleen *yang.*

The major symptom complexes produced by pathogenic dampness are summarized in table 5.4.

Dryness

Dryness is the characteristic climate factor in autumn. In this season, lack of moisture causes many objects in nature to dry out, wrinkle, crack, and wither. The pathological effects of diseases of dryness are analogous to these effects of the autumn climate. They can be recognized by the following characteristics:

DISEASES OF DRYNESS DEPLETE FLUIDS IN THE BODY, CAUSING SENSATIONS OF DRYNESS.

Dryness is a *yang* pathogenic factor. It tends to exhaust the fluids of the body, causing dryness of the mouth, nose, throat, lips, and tongue. Fluid depletion also leads to dry and chapped skin, lustreless hair, constipation, and scanty urine.

DISEASES OF DRYNESS ATTACK THE LUNG AND THE KIDNEY.

By impairing the fluid of the lung, pathogenic dryness may lead to a failure of the disseminating function of the lung, with accompanying symptoms of lung dryness. Since the lung and large intestine are related *zang-fu* organs, the attack on the lung may also dis-

TABLE 5.5. Symptom-Complexes of Pathogenic Dryness

Exogenous Dryness (Warm)
Pathogenic dryness that originates in hot weather is marked by fever; a slight aversion to wind and cold; a dry, hot feeling in the nose; headache, hypohidrosis; thirst; restlessness; dry cough with little expectoration or expectoration of bloody sputum; and difficulty in coughing. The pulse is floating, choppy, and rapid.

Exogenous Dryness (Cool)
This symptom-complex occurs most commonly in the autumn when the weather becomes cool. Its symptoms include a marked aversion to cold, fever, anhidrosis, headache, nasal obstruction, dryness of the mouth and throat, and a dry cough with little expectoration. The pulse is floating and choppy.

Endogenous Dryness
This symptom-complex results from a severe insufficiency of body fluid. It is called the symptom-complex of "insufficiency of fluids" or "dryness of blood." Its symptoms are dryness of the mouth and throat, dry and rough skin, lustreless and withered hair, emaciation, scanty urine and dryness of stools. The pulse is deep, thready, and choppy.

turb the transporting function of the large intestine, producing constipation.

Kidney *yin* is the origin of the fluids of the five organs. Exogenous pathogenic dryness—brought about by the lack of moisture in periods of dry weather or in the surrounding environment—exhausts the fluid which, in turn, creates a condition of insufficiency of kidney *yin.*

Similarly, insufficient vital essence in either the kidney or lung produces endogenous pathogenic dryness.

Table 5.5 reviews the major symptom-complexes of pathogenic dryness.

Fire

A surplus of *qi* may bring on fire symptoms.

Yin deficiency gives rise to interior heat, while a preponderance of *yang* causes exterior heat.

"Treatise on the Regulation of Channels" in
Simple Questions

Fire, like heat, has its source in hot conditions. But while heat is strictly a seasonal pathogenic factor, occurring only in summerlike weather, diseases caused by pathogenic fire may occur in any season. The distinguishing features of such diseases are as follows:

IN DISEASES OF FIRE, SYMPTOMS APPEAR PRIMARILY IN THE HEAD.

Fire is a *yang* pathogenic factor. Its characteristic motion is to flare up, and diseases of pathogenic fire therefore tend to display symptoms of exuberant fire in the head, on the face, and in the sense organs. Flaring up of fire in the heart, for example, produces ulcers in the mouth and on the tongue. Flaring up of fire in the stomach leads to swollen and painful gums. Excess fire in the liver can be recognized by a feeling of distension and pain in the head as well as painful, swollen, and pink eyes.

Diseases of fire have symptoms of dryness. Pathogenic fire burns vital essence, producing dryness. Thus, in addition to symptoms of heat, diseases of fire have symptoms of dryness: thirst, dryness of the mouth and throat, constipation, and concentrated urine.

FIRE DISEASES OFTEN LEAD TO DISEASES OF ENDOGENOUS WIND.

As exogenous pathogenic heat invades the body, it may burn the Liver Channel and impair fluids, producing malnutrition of the tendons and vessels and stirring up endogenous wind in the liver. In Chinese traditional medical thought, this is known as "extreme heat stirring up wind." The symptoms are high fever, coma and delirium, convulsions, a tendency for the eyes to roll back, rigidity of the neck, and opisthotonus.

FIRE DISEASES MAY INVOLVE HEMORRHAGING.

Accelerated blood circulation is a characteristic feature of diseases of pathogenic fire, since warmth generates the flow of blood and exuberant pathogenic fire greatly speeds up blood flow. An extremely rapid blood flow, in turn, often impairs the vessels, causing various forms of hemorrhaging, including hematemesis, epistaxis, hematochezia, and hematuria.

TABLE 5.6. Symptom-Complexes of Pathogenic Fire

Exogenous Fire

This symptom-complex is typical of infectious disease, particularly when the *qi* (secondary defensive), *ying* (nutrient), and *xue* (blood) systems are involved. Symptoms are high fever, intolerance of heat, profuse sweating, anxiety, thirst, and a preference for cold beverages. In severe cases, symptoms may include mania, loss of consciousness, delirium, and stirring up of endogenous wind or bleeding. The pulse is overflowing and rapid.

Endogenous Fire (Preponderant *Yang*)

Endogenous fire results from a disharmony of *yin* and *yang*, in the *zang-fu* organs. If the imbalance results from preponderant *yang*, the heart, liver, lung, and stomach are affected. Symptoms include ulcers of the mouth and tongue, pink eyes, a bitter taste in the mouth, anxiety, a dry and sore throat, expectoration of yellow sputum or purulent blood, swollen and painful gums, thirst, a preference for cold beverages, constipation, and concentrated urine. The pulse is rapid.

Endogenous Fire (Deficient *Yin*)

If endogenous fire results from deficient *yin*, the organs affected are the lung, kidney, heart, and liver. Symptoms include a feverish sensation in the chest, palms, and soles, insomnia and night sweats, dryness of the throat and eyes, dizziness, and ringing in the ears. The pulse is thready and rapid.

FIRE DISEASES MAY RESULT FROM ANY OF THE OTHER FIVE EXCESSES.

Under certain conditions, any of the other five excesses—wind, cold, heat, dampness and dryness—may transform into pathogenic fire. The "seven emotions," which are the principal endogenous pathogenic factors and which will be described below, may also turn into pathogenic fire.

The characteristic symptom-complexes of pathogenic fire appear in table 5.6.

THE SEVEN EMOTIONS: THE SOURCE OF INTERNAL DISORDER

Rage causes *qi* to flow upward; joy allows *qi* to be relaxed; grief produces dejected *qi;* terror causes *qi* to decend; fright drives *qi* to disorder; and pensiveness makes *qi* stagnate.

"Treatise on Abrupt Pains" in *Plain Questions*

In traditional Chinese medicine, emotions are the principal endogenous source of disease. Emotions have a material basis: the essential *qi* of the five organs constitutes this material basis. Emotional activities are therefore closely related to the functioning of the internal organs. In fact, emotions find expression only when the internal organs respond to various external stimuli.[3]

Under ordinary conditions, emotions are normal reactions to external stimuli. "Being joyful, angry, sorry, and gay are natural emotions for human beings," says traditional Chinese medicine. Without these emotions, disease would occur. However, if emotional excitation is extremely abrupt or intense, or if it is persistent and exceeds the normal endurance of the human body, emotions may produce functional disorders of the *zang-fu* organs, impeding the harmonious balance of *yin* and *yang, qi* and blood. The emotions then become pathogenic factors, producing disease and organic lesions. They are classified as "endogenous injuries" since the diseases they cause originate in the interior of the body and directly affect the related internal organs.[4]

According to traditional Chinese medicine, there are seven basic emotions. These are: joy, anger, sadness, pensiveness, grief, fear, and fright. Each of these emotions corresponds to a particular *zang* organ.[5] Rage, for example, is said to injure the liver; excessive fear disrupts the kidney, and so on. However, the heart has a special role to play in the development of disease from the seven emotions. The heart, as explained in chapter 3, houses consciousness; it governs all the five *zang* and six *fu* organs. Therefore, extreme emotional stimuli will first attack the heart, and only subsequently the corresponding internal organs.

3. While the emotions are classified as "endogenous pathogenic factors," they are also related to external circumstance. Thus traditional Chinese medicine states that emotions, being reflections of the human attitude toward numerous external stimuli and phenomena and developed through mental activities, are social in nature. Thus, the emotions of a person living in society and participating in social activities are bound to be influenced by social factors.

4. Emotions have a broader meaning in Chinese medicine than in Western science. In traditional Chinese medical thought, emotions are closely related to the functioning of the internal organs. Mental disorders may injure the internal organs, while functional disturbances of the internal organs may also find their reflection mentally.

5. While there are seven emotions and five *zang* organs, two of the *zang* organs—the heart and lung—each have an additional emotion associated with them. This is further explained in the text.

The seven emotions cause disease by disrupting the normal ascending and descending flow of *qi*. As the above quote from *Plain Questions* suggests, different emotions produce different pathological changes in the flow of *qi*. Such dysfunctions of *qi* will, in turn, produce a dysfunction in the flow of blood. Ultimately, these disorders of *qi* and blood affect the *zang-fu* organs directly.

The reverse is also true. A functional disorder of the internal organs may lead to a preponderance or stagnation of *qi*. This disruption of the normal flow of *qi* may readily produce abnormal emotions: liver trouble often produces irritability; patients with heart problems will frequently laugh or weep for no apparent reason.

Like the six excesses, the seven emotions each represent a specific symptom-complex. These are as follows:

Joy

Joy is the emotional expression of the heart. When one is joyful and happy, his spirits are high and he is cheerful. When normal, this emotion is actually beneficial to the body, for it encourages the circulation of *qi* and blood. However, over-joy produces adverse effects primarily on the heart, although the lung may also be affected since both organs are situated in the upper burner. The symptom-complex caused by over-joy is a scattering of heart *qi* resulting in inability to concentrate.

Anger

Anger is most closely linked to the liver. It causes an adverse flow of liver *qi,* interrupts the regular circulation of *qi* and blood, and may also cause stagnation of *qi*. Since the lung governs the *qi* of the entire body, the adverse flow of liver *qi* may cause an upward adverse flow of lung *qi*. Pathogenic anger, then, produces a functional disharmony of the liver and lung.

The symptom-complex associated with pathogenic anger includes dizziness, headache, flushed or livid face, reddened eyes, a bitter taste in the mouth, dryness of the throat, a sensation of a foreign body in the throat, distending pain in the ribs, a feeling of suffocation, frequent sighing, irritability, mental depression, and—in women—menstrual irregularities and distending pain or lumps in the breast. The disruption of the regular circulation of blood and *qi* may lead to loss of consciousness; the adverse flow of lung *qi* can cause choking. The pulse is wiry, drawn tight like a bowstring.

Sadness

Excessive sadness or melancholy takes its toll primarily on the lung. It impedes the normal flow of lung *qi* and causes its stagnation. Symptoms are usually a feeling of oppression in the chest and depression.

Protracted stagnation of lung *qi* may transform into fire which, in turn, impairs the vital essence of the lung. It may also harm the spleen, disturbing its digestive function and the ability to absorb nutrients and water. Typical symptoms are lack of appetite, restlessness, insomnia, and emaciation.

Pensiveness

Excessive pensiveness injures the spleen. It causes depression and ultimately stagnation of *qi,* resulting in a failure of the spleen and stomach in transporting nutrients and water throughout the body. Loss of appetite is the most common symptom.

While pensiveness attacks the spleen, it is said to originate from the heart, since it "occupies one's hearing and makes one's mind concentrate." Prolonged pensiveness may therefore cause stagnation of *qi* in both the heart and spleen, leading to symptoms of heart disease. These symptoms include depression, anxiety, weakness of the limbs, poor appetite, abdominal distension, restless sleep, amnesia, continuous violent palpitations, and—in severe cases—dementia. In women, menstrual irregularities often occur.

If stagnation of *qi* of the heart and spleen continues, a symptom-complex known as "depressed heat in the heart and spleen" appears. This symptom-complex includes insomnia, anxiety, palpitations, a tendency to be easily startled, dryness of the mouth and lips, ulceration of the mouth and tongue, a yellow coating on the tongue with a reddened tongue tip, loss of appetite, and constipation. The pulse is usually deep and rapid.

Grief

Extreme grief also injures the lung. Since the lung controls the *qi* of the entire body, grief may lead to a dejection or stagnation of *qi*. The result is hypofunctioning of the internal organs. The common symptoms are pallor, difficulty in breathing, a sensation of suffocation in the chest, listlessness, depression, reticence, sighing, loss of appetite, and difficulty in urination and defecation.

Fear

Fear is an extension of timidity that arises spontaneously within the body. It is due to the hypofunctioning of the internal organs. Extreme fear injures the kidney, causing the normal upward flow of kidney *qi* to reverse itself and flow downward. The resulting symptoms include a desire for solitude, listlessness, soreness in the lumbar region and feebleness of the lower limbs, inability to control urination and defecation, and bedwetting. In women, menstrual periods will be long and irregular. The pulse is deep and thready.

Fright

Fright is a state of panic aroused by a sudden external event. Fright affects the heart the most, and produces a general dysfunction of *qi;* as a result, heart *qi* is said to "wander about, adhering to nothing." Clinical manifestations of this emotion include a tendency to be easily startled, sudden palpitations or continual violent palpitations, and mental restlessness.

NEITHER EXOGENOUS NOR ENDOGENOUS: PESTILENCE, INJURY, AND LIFE-STYLE

Traditionally, the causes of disease have been put into three categories: exogenous, endogenous, and "neither exogenous nor endogenous." The exogenous factors were the six excesses or climatic factors. The endogenous factors were the seven emotions. But there remained several causes of illness that could not be classified as climatic or emotional; these were called "neither exogenous nor endogenous."

Today, traditional Chinese practitioners often speak of only two classes of pathogenic factors—exogenous and endogenous. In addition to the six excesses, they view pestilence, traumatic injuries, insect or animal bites, and parasitic infection as exogenous factors. In addition to the seven emotions, they classify irregular diet, excess of sexual activity or physical exertion, and conditions of excess phlegm and stagnant blood as endogenous factors. In Chinese medicine, these pathogenic factors are explained as follows.

Pestilence

Traditional Chinese medicine has always recognized epidemic noxious factors as a cause of disease. These factors include the bacteria and viruses of modern epidemiology. Pestilential diseases are characterized by their swift onset, their consistency of symptoms, and their high level of infectiousness. They tend to be fatal in severe cases. They may occur in scattered cases or spread as an epidemic, endangering life.

Traumatic Injuries, Insect and Animal Bites, and Parasitic Infections

Another class of exogenous pathogenic factors includes all traumatic injuries, insect and animal bites, and parasitic diseases. Traumatic injuries are those resulting from external mechanical violence: gunshot injuries, cuts, injuries from falls, contusions, strains, burns, and frostbite. In mild cases, such injuries may cause skin and muscle wounds, bleeding, pain, swelling, and bruises; severe cases produce injuries to the tendons, bones, and internal organs; dislocations; fractures; and compression or even rupture of the internal organs. Such wounds may become infected by bacteria.

If infection occurs—or if the injuries affect vital organs—massive hemorrhaging is likely, and serious pathological changes such as coma, shock, and toxic convulsions may appear. Frostbite causes a local stagnation of blood, leading to a drop in body temperature and an inflammation of the hands and feet.

In mild cases, bites by insects, reptiles, and animals (including rabid dogs) may cause bleeding, bruises, and pain. Severe cases exhibit a syndrome of general poisoning due to toxins circulating in the blood. Such poisoning may result in fever, convulsions, coma, or manic insanity.

Intestinal parasites such as ascarids, pinworms, hookworms, cestodes, and fasciolopsis often cause abdominal pain, a sallow face, and anal itching. Those afflicted frequently have cravings for particular foods. Traditional Chinese medicine also recognizes a symptom-complex known as "acute abdominal pain with cold limbs due to ascarids." As its name implies, this complex is characterized by severe pain in the stomach and cold limbs. It corresponds to the biliary ascariasis of Western medicine. Finally, there are the blood parasites known as *schistosomes*. Symptoms of schistosomiasis include a disturbance in the blood circulation and, in severe cases, stagnation of blood with retention of water in the abdomen.

Irregular Diet

Irregular food intake is an important pathogenic factor. It can cause injury to the spleen and stomach, leading to their inability to receive, digest, transport, and transform food. Abnormality in the ascending and descending flow of *qi,* blood, and body fluid may also result from such injury; in this case, the resulting accumulation of dampness will produce phlegm, accompanied by symptoms of endogenous heat. Eventually other organs may be affected. Also, irregular food intake may contribute to relapses from serious disease.

Chinese medicine distinguishes three types of dietary irregularities. The first concerns the volume of food. Food should be taken in proper amounts at regular times. Voracious eating as well as too little food intake may lead to disease. Specifically, inadequate food intake leads to malnutrition. If there is insufficient matter for transformation of *qi* and blood, the resulting deficiency condition results in weak vital energy and a lowered body resistance. This condition not only retards development but also leaves the body susceptible to exogenous pathogenic factors.

Excessive eating also injures the stomach and spleen, impairing digestion. The symptoms are distending gastric and abdominal pain, accompanied by a sensation of pressure, loss of appetite, odorous belching, acidic regurgitations, and foul-smelling stools. Excessive food intake in infants may lead to a prolonged accumulation of undigested food which, in turn, may transform into heat and produce phlegm. Extreme dysfunction of the spleen and stomach follow. This condition is known as "infantile malnutrition"; its symptoms include a feverish sensation in the palms, soles, and chest; fullness and distension in the stomach and abdomen; and diarrhea.

The second type of dietary irregularity is the consumption of improper foods. A variety of food should be consumed to assure that the body receives all of the vital nutrients. Personal preferences often lead to diets that are limited in variety; such limited diets may lead to malnutrition and eventually to diseases such as goiter, rickets, night blindness, and beriberi.

Specific foods also produce specific problems. An excess consumption of raw or cold foods injures the function of the stomach and spleen. The resulting deficiency condition is marked by abdominal pain and diarrhea. Pungent or spicy food, taken in excess, impairs the vital essence of the stomach and produces a condition of excess stomach heat. The predominant symptom is a constant feeling of hunger, despite large amounts of food intake. Frequent overeating of very rich foods will produce symptoms of dyspepsia, vertigo, and a sensation of oppression in the chest, as well as carbuncles, ulcers, boils, and internal bleeding, all of which indicate injury to the stomach and spleen.

Alcohol has been recognized for centuries as a food that is likely to produce symptom-complexes of dampness, heat, and phlegm. In the twelfth century, Li Dongyuan wrote a *Treatise on the Spleen and Stomach*. In it, he referred to a disease called "alcoholics," which was defined as chronic pathological lumps in the stomach due to indulgence in alcoholic beverages. The symptoms of emaciation, accumulation of water in the abdomen, and abdominal masses are similar to those of modern medicine's alcoholic cirrhosis.

The third dietary irregularity results from the consumption of spoiled or unsanitary food. This is a common cause of gastrointestinal illness as well as infectious diseases of the alimentary tract. The typical symptoms include distending pain in the abdomen, nausea, vomiting, agitation of the intestinal tract, diarrhea, the sensation of needing to defecate, and dysentery.

Excessive Sexual Activity and Physical Exertion

Excessive sexual activity and overexertion are also endogenous pathogenic factors. Excessive sexual activity consumes essence and kidney *qi,* leading to a deficiency condition. The result is a general debility, with aching and weakness in the lumbar region and knee joints, dizziness, ringing in the ears, listlessness and lassitude. In men, the condition is often accompanied by nocturnal emissions, spermatorrhea, and impotency. In women, menstrual irregularities and foul-smelling vaginal discharges are typical.

Overexertion produces a deficiency of original *qi* and hypofunctioning of the *zang-fu* organs, giving rise to general debility. In this case, the symptoms are feebleness, general sluggishness, lassitude, apathy, and asthma brought on by activity. The pathology here often includes loss of blood in the heart. (The latter is also commonly seen in cases of intense mental work or excessive pensiveness.) The loss of heart blood produces palpitations, amnesia, insomnia, and dream-disturbed sleep. On the other hand, inadequate physical work and exercise may also result in a deficiency of vital energy and a lowered body resistance, since the circulation of blood and *qi* is slow. Symptoms of this type of deficiency are poor appetite, lassitude, feebleness of the limbs, listlessness, vertigo, palpitations, and a secondary illness elicited by these conditions.

Retention of Phlegm and Fluid

Queer diseases are caused by retention of phlegm and fluid, which is the source of all disorders.
"The Causes of Miscellenous Diseases" in *Shen's*
Work on the Importance of Life Preservation

When organs of the body do not function properly, they produce two pathological substances: phlegm and stagnant blood. These substances may induce various secondary diseases by acting either directly or indirectly on certain parts of the body or on certain internal organs.

Phlegm and retained fluid refer, in a broad sense, to diseases caused by a disturbance of water metabolism in the body and by the accumulation of fluids in the body cavity and extremities. In a narrow sense, these terms label a disease of water retention in the stomach and intestines. Its main manifestations are dizziness, nausea, vomiting, shortness of breath, palpitations, manic insanity, and loss of consciousness.

Water is the source of phlegm and retained fluid. Chinese medicine states that accumulated water transforms into morbid fluid, condensation of which turns into phlegm. Phlegm thus develops as a secondary pathogen when the body's water metabolism is disturbed by pathogenic water-dampness. Functional disturbances of the *qi* of the lung, spleen, and kidney are usually at fault; but retained phlegm and fluid may also appear when the passages of the Triple Burners are blocked and the normal transport, distribution, and excretion of body fluid are therefore interrupted.

Pathogenic phlegm may accumulate anywhere in the body, either in the internal organs or superficially in the tendons, bones, skin, and muscles. In general, phlegm produces a symptom-complex characterized by visible external signs, such as oozing due to inflammation of the respiratory system, edema, ascites, accumulation of fluids in the tissue surrounding the joints, tubercular abscesses, and tuberculosis of the cervical lymph nodes. It also produces more internal pathological symptoms, such as mental disturbances, accumulations in the thoracic region, intestines, and stomach, and blockage of the channels and collaterals.

Specific problems arise when phlegm accumulates in specific parts of the body. Phlegm that blocks the lung results in coughing with asthmatic breathing and expectoration of sputum. Phlegm in the heart causes dementia, mental confusion, and manic insanity. If the heart channel is obstructed by phlegm, anxiety, a feeling of oppression in the chest, mania, or dementia may appear. Phlegm stagnating in the stomach causes nausea, vomiting, and bloating; subcutaneous accumulation causes phlegmatic limbs, scrofula, and tubercular abscesses.

Phlegm in the channels and collaterals produces numbness of the limbs and partial paralysis. Phlegm in the throat produces the sensation of a foreign body in the throat. Phlegm due to pathogenic wind in the head causes dizziness, nausea, numbness of the limbs, and wheezing with phlegm in the throat. Morbid fluid in the tissues of the skin causes edema. In the costal region, it produces distending pain (especially when the patient coughs or expectorates). If it accumulates in the region above the diaphragm, phlegm causes coughing and difficulty in lying supinely. In the intestines, it produces a sensation of fullness in the chest, poor appetite, and intestinal rumbling.

Stagnant Blood

Like phlegm, stagnant blood is a pathological product that appears when the internal organs fail to function properly. More specifically, stagnant blood accumulates when the flow of blood is irregular due to deficiency of *qi* or when it is attacked by pathogenic cold. Internal hemmorrhaging as a result of pathogenic heat or traumatic injuries may also create stagnant blood. This blood coagulates, further obstructing the flow of *qi* and blood and impeding normal regeneration. Also, once it becomes stagnant, it loses its natural ability to nourish and moisten the body and, instead, becomes harmful to it.

Unlike phlegm, stagnant blood and the diseases it produces appear in a fixed location in the body. The symptoms of stagnant blood depend on the location. For example,

—Stagnancy in the lung produces pain in the chest and expectoration of blood.

—Stagnant blood in the stomach and intestines causes hematemesis and hematochezia.

—In the liver, it produces pain and lumps or masses in the costal region.

—In the uterus, stagnant blood results in pain in the lower abdomen, menstrual irregularities, dysmenorrhea, amenorrhea, uterine bleeding, and menstruation with dark purple blood and clots.

—Stagnation of blood in the limbs causes swelling and pain in the muscles and blue skin.

While the symptoms of stagnant blood vary with location in the body, there are some symptoms common to all cases of stagnant blood. Since the accumulation of stagnant blood can be viewed as a foreign object in the body, it will readily produce pain. Typically, this pain will be a sensation of stabbing or incising in a fixed area, and it will be aggravated by pressure. A lack of oxygen due to poor blood circulation produces a blue coloration of the skin and a dark purple tongue. The failure of *qi* and blood circulation results in masses or lumps. As stagnant blood blocks the flow of blood, vessels are broken, and hemorrhaging or bruising appears. Protracted stagnancy means that new blood is not regenerated; in this case, malnutrition leads to external symptoms of scaly dry skin. The pulse in cases of blood stagnation is fine, choppy, or intermittent and irregular.

IN SUMMARY

Traditional Chinese medicine divides the causes of disease into two principal categories: exogenous and endogenous.

Exogenous causes are environmental and are usually related to climatic conditions. The most common exogenous pathogenic factors are known as the "Six Excesses"; they include wind, cold, heat, dampness, dryness, and fire.

The main endogenous causes of disease are the "Seven Emotions." In Chinese medicine, the essential *qi* of the *zang* organs are the material basis of emotions. An extreme emotion can thus impair the *zang-fu* organs; similarly, a dysfunction of one of the organs can lead to abnormal emotions. The Seven Emotions are joy, anger, sadness, pensiveness, grief, fear, and fright.

Each of the Six Excesses and the Seven Emotions affects a specific *zang* organ. Accordingly, if the cause of the illness is known, the location of the disease can be determined. Conversely, if the location is known, the cause can usually be deduced.

At the same time, neither the organs of the body nor the pathogenic factors act in isolation. One pathogenic factor can generate another, and one diseased organ can weaken another. The path of disease is therefore variable, as chapter 6 will demonstrate.

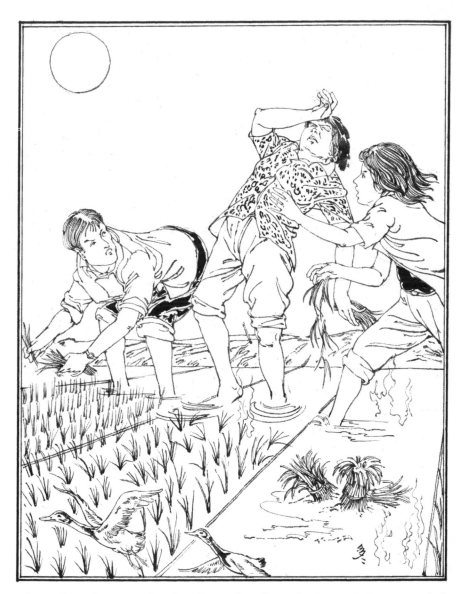

A rural worker experiencing discomfort from the heat of the sun and the coldness of the water.

CHAPTER SIX

Pathogenesis:
The Course of Disease

THE TRADITIONAL CHINESE theory of etiology described in the last chapter is a theory of the causes and conditions of disease: climatic factors, emotions, pestilence, trauma, diet, excesses of lifestyle, and pathological products of the body's own metabolism.

These pathogenic factors are, however, only the conditions under which disease occurs. By themselves, they determine neither the onset of disease nor its outcome. To describe the laws that govern the onset, development, and outcome of disease is the realm of the theory of pathogenesis.

According to Chinese medicine, the body has a series of self-adjusting systems. As explained in chapter 2, these systems operate according to the basic principles of the theory of *yin* and *yang*. They work to balance the functions of the *zang-fu* organs and channels, *qi* and blood, body fluid, and tissues. They also allow the body to maintain its normal functions while adapting to a constantly changing external environment.

Disease occurs when the dynamic equilibrium within the body and between the body and environment fails, damaging the normal physiological functions to the point that there is:

• an imbalance between *yin* and *yang*
• a derangement of *qi* and blood

• a disturbance in the ascending and descending functions of the organs

Because the body has the ability for self-adjustment, two processes come into play at every stage of disease: (1) pathogenic factors damage the body; and (2) the body's self-defense system is mobilized against the damage. The course of disease is thus a contest between pathogenic factors and what Chinese medicine calls "antipathogenic *qi* (or the antipathogenic factor)." The path of any specific disease cannot be known without an understanding of the general laws that govern these two processes.

THE CONTEST BETWEEN PATHOGENIC AND ANTIPATHOGENIC *QI*

A preponderance of the antipathogenic factor in the interior of the body protects the individual from the invasion of the pathogenic factor.

"Treatise on Acupuncture" in the
Addendum to Plain Questions

When the pathogenic factor invades, the antipathogenic factor is weak.

"Treatise on Fevers" in *Plain Questions*

Keep strong, and disease will find no way to attack.

Synopsis of the Golden Chamber

The human body has the ability to resist the invasion of pathogenic factors and to repair itself when those factors cause it harm. This ability is known as antipathogenic *qi.*

According to traditional Chinese medicine, the history of a disease is the history of the relationship between antipathogenic *qi* and the pathogenic factor or factors. In its simplest form, this relationship is a struggle—a struggle between opposites.

In the course of this struggle, antipathogenic *qi* wages its battle by adjusting the balance between *yin* and *yang*, between blood and *qi,* and between the ascending and descending functions of the organs. When antipathogenic *qi* is vigorous and the pathogenic factor is weak, these adjustments are adequate, and the invasion of the pathogenic factor is hindered. Even if the invasion succeeds, it will not necessarily produce disease as long as antipathogenic *qi* prevails. For this reason, *Chinese medicine views antipathogenic qi as the primary factor in the occurrence of disease, while the pathogenic factor is only the conditional factor.*[1]

The pattern of the struggle between antipathogenic *qi* and pathogenic factors is the universal struggle between *yin* and *yang*, between deficiency and excess. In general, a rise in antipathogenic *qi* leads to a consuming of the pathogenic factors; conversely, a rise in the pathogenic factor leads to a consuming of antipathogenic *qi*. (See chapter 2.)

As the struggle proceeds, symptom-complexes appear. These will be symptom-complexes of excess or deficiency:

> Excess implies preponderance of the pathogenic factor, while deficiency points to a loss of vital energy.
>
> "Treatise on Deficiency and Excess"
> in *Plain Questions*

A symptom-complex of excess means that the pathogenic factor is preponderant. In the conflict taking place in the body, the pathogenic factor is hyperactive, but the antipathogenic *qi* is still strong, and physiological functions are not impaired. The result is a severe struggle that is characteristic of the early stages of disease caused either by the six exogenous pathogenic factors or by improper food intake, excessive phlegm, and stagnant blood or body fluid.

A symptom-complex of deficiency appears when antipathogenic *qi* is impaired. (For a description of the factors that determine the strength of antipathogenic *qi*, see the next section.) In this case, physiological functioning is weak, and blood and essence are deficient. This type of symptom-complex occurs most commonly in the advanced stage of a disease or in the course of various chronic diseases.

The relationship between pathogenic and antipathogenic factors is constantly changing. Accordingly, a symptom-complex of excess may be transformed into one of deficiency. Acute disease or diseases caused by stagnation of *qi* or blood are characterized primarily by a short course and rapid development in which the pathogenic factor is pre-

---

1. Chinese medicine, of course, does not deny the important role of exogenous pathogenic factors in bringing about disease, especially in cases of epidemic disease. In fact, the "Treatise on Acupuncture" in the *Addendum to Plain Questions* warns that "apart from maintaining a strong body resistance, epidemic disease agents must be kept away from the body." However, antipathogenic *qi* is the decisive factor.

ponderant. If such a disease is not treated or if the therapy fails, the pathogenic factors will remain in the body, injuring the antipathogenic *qi*. The original symptom-complex of excess will then transform into one of deficiency or a complicated condition of both deficiency and excess.

Chronic diseases, by contrast, begin as deficiency conditions and have a more protracted development. If they are not treated or if therapy fails—if antipathogenic *qi* is too weak to overcome the pathogenic factors—the symptom-complex of deficiency will transform into a condition of both excess and deficiency. The symptoms of this condition include retention of phlegm, food, blood, and fluids, which leads to a blockage of the passageways.[2]

The transformation of excess and deficiency is a critical development in the course of diseases. Without an understanding of this process of change, the practitioner is liable to make mistakes in the differentiation of symptom-complexes and hence fail to understand the true nature of a disease.

ANTIPATHOGENIC *QI:* WEAK OR STRONG?

Four main factors determine whether antipathogenic *qi* is weak or strong:

Constitution

Different people have different physical constitutions. Chinese medicine, like Western science, recognizes the role of both inheritance and environment in determining the constitution of any given individual. They distinguish between the so-called "former heaven" and the "latter heaven."

The "former heaven" refers to qualities inherited from one's parents. It is one's "natural endowment." Already at the moment of

2. A type of consumptive disease found in women, usually characterized by retarded menstrual flow, recurrent low fever, and general debility, is an example of a deficiency condition that has transformed into a condition of both deficiency and excess: consumption with blood stasis.

birth, this "former heaven" has begun to shape the course of future disease in an individual:

> Those who differ in their natural endowment have different dispositions, either firm or gentle; they have different constitutions, either weak or strong; and they have different heights, either tall or short. Their physiological and pathological changes vary with the *yin* and *yang* of this natural endowment.
>
> "Treatise on Life Span and the Firm or Gentle
> Disposition" in *Miraculous Pivot*

Nutrition

The "latter heaven" refers to qualities that are acquired in the course of life, principally as a result of nutrition. Excess weight and emaciation can both be primary causes of disease. But even beyond these extremes, different types of physiques—which result from different patterns of diet—will point to the most likely patterns of disease. These patterns of disease are patterns of excess and deficiency of *yin* and *yang*. For example, those with a heavy physique are inclined to be deficient in *yang;* they will suffer from excess dampness and phlegm. They are also likely to experience diseases of pathogenic cold as a result of harmful *yin*. People with emaciated physiques are more likely to be deficient in *yin;* they will have symptoms of preponderant liver *qi* and excess fire and heat. Women may also be more inclined to *yin* deficiency, by constitution, than men.

Mental State

Mental state also influences the strength of antipathogenic *qi*. In traditional Chinese medicine, mental state always influences the functioning of *qi* and blood. Mental state may thus become an endogenous pathogenic factor, or it may induce disorders of the organs, *qi,* and blood, which in turn lead to disease. Certain types of mental stimulation also weaken antipathogenic *qi,* allowing the invasion of other pathogenic factors. Prolonged depression, in particular, produces insomnia, loss of appetite, dysfunctions of the organs, blockages in the flow of *qi* and blood, and lowered body resistance. These are favorable conditions for an attack by pathogenic factors.

Poor Habits

Habits of all sorts may also weaken the body's resistance. For example, persistent staring is said to impair blood. Continual sleeping impairs *qi*. Long periods of sitting, standing, and walking weaken the muscles, bones, and tendons, respectively. Excessive mental work may injure the heart and spleen. Identifying such habits is thus of vital importance in the diagnosis, prevention, and treatment of occupational illnesses, in particular.

WHEN ANTIPATHOGENIC *QI* FAILS

Recovery from a disease means that antipathogenic *qi* has prevailed over the pathogenic factor. The course of the disease has been one in which the preponderant antipathogenic *qi*—the strong body resistance—has been able to check the growth of the pathogenic factor. The attack has probably been mild, and the duration of the disease short. The normal functioning of the *zang-fu* organs and of *qi* and blood has resumed, and the relative equilibrium of *yin* and *yang* is reestablished on a new basis.

The opposite process, of course, results in deterioration.

In any disease, deterioration occurs when the pathogenic factor overwhelms antipathogenic *qi*. The latter gradually declines. Also, additional disorders in the functioning of the organs, *qi,* and blood may appear. These weaknesses lead ultimately to continuous damage by the pathogenic factor, and the patient's condition deteriorates.

Three factors indicate the advance of illness. The first is the appearance of *interior* symptom-complexes: abdominal distension, constipation, or diarrhea are typical symptoms indicating this development. In the first stages of a disease, most of the symptoms will be *exterior* symptoms or those involving the body surface. If these disappear, but the interior symptoms replace them, the body's condition has worsened.[3]

3. By contrast, Chinese medicine says that "when the interior symptoms exit from the interior," recovery usually results. Measles provides an example. Initially, the eruption of papules is hindered because the papula toxin is active in the interior of the body, producing overly abundant internal heat. If the disease is treated with a medicine that brings out the papules, the eruptions are induced and the papula toxin is expelled from the interior. This is the recession of the disease from the interior to the body surface, which indicates that recovery is likely.

The second indication of the advance of illness is the development of *cold* symptom-complexes. In cases of prolonged disease, the defeat of antipathogenic *qi* leads to damage to the body's heat. The result is that the *heat* symptom-complexes that often appear in the initial stages of a disease are replaced by cold symptom-complexes, marked by low fever and chills.

The appearance of symptom-complexes of *deficiency* is the third indicator that the disease has advanced. If signs of excess are replaced by signs of deficiency or a mixture of excess and deficiency, the body's condition has deteriorated.

If treatment is delayed in these advanced stages, the pathogenic factor becomes rampant, antipathogenic *qi* grows extremely weak, and the functional activities of the *zang-fu* organs, *qi,* and blood verge on failure. Life ends, according to traditional Chinese medicine, when *"yin* and *yang* part and *qi* and blood run out."

In the losing struggle between antipathogenic *qi* and the pathogenic factor, a train of pathological changes occurs. The body's internal environment becomes imbalanced. In particular, the balance between *yang* and *yin* is disrupted. Dysfunctions of *qi* and blood appear, and the normal ascending and descending movement of the *qi* of the *zang-fu* organs becomes disturbed. The theory of pathogenesis of traditional Chinese medicine states that no matter how complicated the symptom-complexes may appear or how volatile the condition is, the fundamental pathological process is nothing more than an imbalance between *yin* and *yang,* a derangement of *qi,* and an obstruction of the flow of *qi* from the organs.[4]

THE FAILURE OF *YANG*

All illness is the result of an imbalance of *yin* and *yang.* In the body, this imbalance appears as a disorder of either *yang qi* or *yin* essence.

4. An important research task is to explore more completely the nature of the imbalance of *yin* and *yang,* the derangement of *qi* and blood, and the disturbances in the upward and downward flow of *qi* from the standpoint of function, metabolism, and structure. It has been argued that the "Eight Guiding Principles" used to distinguish symptom-complexes are based not only on physiology and biochemistry, but also on pathoanatomy. Much current research in China is directed toward establishing the material basis of the symptom-complexes and the Eight Guiding Principles from the point of view of pathophysiology and pathoanatomy.

As explained in chapter 3, *yang qi* is the body's vital energy. Its main function is to warm and defend the body, to nourish the nerves, and to promote metabolism as well as the activities of the *zang-fu* organs. It initiates all physiological activities and thereby maintains the life processes.

Yin essence—or vital essence—is the material counterpart to vital energy. It includes such substances as blood and body fluid, which provide the material foundation for life's activities. Vital essence is said to moisten the internal organs and the interstitial spaces between the skin and the flesh. It is also said to "whet" the spirit. It gives rise to vital energy.

Under normal conditions, vital energy and vital essence are continuously consuming and reproducing each other. Vital energy moves upward, producing heat and motion. Vital essence moves downward, producing cold and quiescence. When the patterns of ascending and descending, assembly and dispersion, movement and quiescence are balanced, there is a harmonious equilibrium of normal physiological activities. Imbalance occurs when either vital energy or vital essence fails.

Vital energy can fail in five ways:

IF *YANG* BECOMES PREPONDERANT. *Yang* becomes preponderant either when pathogenic heat attacks the body or when pathogenic cold invades the interior of the body and is transformed into heat (since cold is of a *yin* nature and heat is of a *yang* nature). Preponderant *yang* may also be the result of pathogenic fire that arises from persistent abnormal emotions or from long-standing obstruction of *qi* or from blood stasis.

Preponderant *yang* means that the organs, tissues, and other body systems are hyperfunctioning. Metabolism is excessively vigorous. The individual is overly excitable and overreacts to stimuli. There is an excess of heat.

This condition is known in traditional Chinese medicine as a "heat symptom-complex due to excessive pathogenic factors." It is characterized by fever and the consumption of body fluid. It eventually impairs vital essence.[5]

5. Current efforts made by Dr. Kuang Tiaoyuan in his *Study on Pathology by Traditional Chinese Medicine* (Shanghai Science and Technology Press, 1980, p. 106) describe this condition in Western terms: "There is acute inflammation. Cells become swollen, degenerated,

IF YANG BECOMES DEFICIENT. A deficiency of *yang* usually stems from an innate insufficiency, from postnatal malnutrition, or from an impairment of *yang* by a long illness. In these cases, an insufficiency of "fire in the vital gate"[6] means a reduction of heat production or hypofunction of the organs, leading to failure of *yang* to check *yin*. The body is thus subjected to a preponderance of cold and fluid retention in its interior.

Yang deficiency is characterized by hypofunctioning of the organs, tissues, and other body systems. Responsiveness and metabolism decline. Physiological activities are weak, body resistance is low, and there is insufficient heat.

This condition produces a symptom-complex of exterior cold. It is marked by pallor, an aversion to cold, and a tendency for the extremities to be cold. A person in this condition is susceptible to catching colds. A symptom-complex of cold may also lead to a disturbance in the process of water metabolism, causing dampness and stagnation of fluid. Eventually, it will impede the generation of *yin* and lead to insufficient generation of vital essence.[7]

and necrotic. Blood vessels vasodilate due to congestion. These conditions are accompanied by an excessive inflammatory effusion that includes neutrophilic leukocytes. Occasionally, acute suppurative inflammation occurs. There is a rise in either local or systemic temperatures, a loss of large amounts of body fluid, an increase in blood concentration, and a compensatory increase in heart rate. This results from the accumulation of bacterial toxins and metabolic products."

Also typical is a disturbance in blood circulation, with either arterial congestion or hemorrhaging. Traditional Chinese medicine states that blood is forced to escape from the vessels when there is an invasion of *ying* and *xue* systems by pathogenic heat.

6. See the description of the kidney in chapter 3.

7. Recent Chinese studies suggest that the condition described as *yang* deficiency includes the following: degeneration and atrophy of the endocrine glands in common. (Since the endocrine glands play an important role in regulating metabolism, it is not surprising that this kind of disorder affects the functioning of the entire body.) In addition, atrophy and degeneration of a variety of cell types has been observed. Degeneration of the renal, hepatic, and cerebral cells, accompanied by conditions of turbidity, swelling, and fat degeneration, are common in various chronic consumptive diseases. This is particularly true of cardiac muscles, in which degeneration of cardiac muscles includes a reduction in cell volume and the precipitation of brown granules at the sides of the cells. This may be the main reason for the hypofunctioning of the cardiovascular system when the pulse is weak and feeble.

Also found in this symptom-complex are changes due to chronic inflammation, especially in cases of severe and prolonged *yang* deficiency. Degeneration, atrophy, and death of the parenchymal cells occurs. These are subsequently replaced by connective tissues, leading ultimately to the malfunctioning of the rest of the organs.

Finally, hypofunctioning of the phagocytic ability of the endothelial system and degeneration of the nervous system have been observed in connection with this symptom-complex.

IF YANG PERISHES. The perishing of *yang* is a serious condition in which *yang* becomes detached from the body substances. It occurs in cases of critical deficiency of *yang* or of disease due to extreme cold. It may also be caused by the escape of *yang* in conditions of excessive perspiration. It appears most commonly in the advanced stages of acute disease, but may also occur in advanced stages of chronic diseases[8] when both vital essence and vital energy are about to be extinguished due to their chronic consumption.

The symptoms that indicate the perishing of *yang* are profuse sweating, a cold sensation of the skin and limbs during inactivity, and a fading pulse—all of which point to the exhaustion of vital energy. Collapse of the body's functional activities is imminent, since the perishing of *yang* leads to a failure in the production of vital essence, which also becomes exhausted. The perishing of *yang* is thus usually followed by the loss of *yin*. Once the interdependent relationship between *yin* and *yang* is destroyed, *yin* becomes divorced from *yang*, and life's activities come to an end.[9]

IF EXCESSIVE YANG HINDERS YIN. Predominant *yang* produces excess heat. If this internal heat is trapped within the body, and *yang* is unable to be released to reach the limbs, traditional Chinese medicine says that "excessive *yang* hinders *yin*."[10] In this state, *yin* and *yang*—and cold and heat—are separated from each other. *Yin* on the exterior of the body becomes disconnected from the overabundant *yang* on the interior. The resulting symptom-complex is one of "true heat and false cold." Its symptoms are normal body heat but cold extremities and a deep pulse.

8. In chronic diseases, this often referred to as the "extinguishing of *yang*."

9. In Western medicine, the symptom-complex of perishing of *yang* is often labeled "shock." Shock—other than traumatic or hemorrhagic shock—has been thought to be related to pathological changes in the heart, lung, or kidney. Recently, however, some Chinese research has indicated that shock is related to the disturbance of the microcirculation and intravascular coagulation mechanisms. (See Kuang Tiaoyuan, *Study on Pathology by Traditional Chinese Medicine,* Shanghai Science and Technology Press, 1980, p. 113.) This explanation is consistent with the clinical symptoms of perishing *yang*: a decrease in effective circulatory blood volume, anoxia in the vital organs, metabolic malfunctioning, and acidosis. These symptoms, in turn, can lead to paralysis, dilation, and coagulation of the minute blood vessels, as well as lowered blood pressure—all of which cause additional difficulties that endanger life.

10. This means that heat inside the body exceeds a maximum value and manifests as false cold externally.

IF *YANG* IS IMPAIRED AND IMPEDES THE GENERATION OF *YIN*. A persistent deficiency of *yang* (vital energy) often leads to impaired generation of *yin* (vital essence). Insufficient essence, in turn, leads eventually to a deficiency of both *yin* and *yang*.

This condition often appears when pathological changes affect any one of the *zang-fu* organs. However, since kidney *yin* and kidney *yang* are the foundation of *yin* and *yang* for all of the *zang* and *fu* organs, the impairment of *yang* that impedes the generation of *yin* in any organ will ultimately create a deficiency of kidney *yang*. If the condition continues, the decrease in the growth of vital essence, together with the constrained function of the kidney, will lead to a deficiency of both *yin* and *yang* of the kidney.

THE FAILURE OF *YIN*

Yin, or vital essence, can also fail in five ways:

IF *YIN* BECOMES PREPONDERANT. A preponderance of *yin* is not an excess or surplus of vital essence. It is rather a disorder of the entire system or of a group of organs and their related systems. In this state, there is an increase in inhibitory processes, a disturbance of metabolism, and an insufficient generation of energy, as well as the accumulation of pathological products such as phlegm. A preponderance of *yin* often appears in cases of deficient *yang,* marked by hypofunctioning of the body.

A preponderance of *yin* is usually the result of exogenous pathogenic factors, such as cold and dampness, that exceed the ability of vital energy to produce warmth. It may also result from a prolonged insufficiency of *yang;* in this case, too, vital energy is insufficient to counter the coagulating effects of cold and dampness. The first condition—that of exogenous cold and dampness—is a case of excess; the second is a condition of both deficiency and excess.

In time, a preponderance of *yin* produces interior cold. The result is a functional inhibition of the internal organs as well as an inhibition of vital energy. Blood does not circulate freely, and there is general hypofunctioning of the system, accompanied by symptoms of cold limbs, stomachache, diarrhea, edema, phlegm, and excessive fluid. This is the symptom-complex of excess cold.[11]

IF *YIN* BECOMES DEFICIENT. When *yin* becomes deficient, both the quantity and quality, of vital essence (including body fluid, essence, and blood) are reduced. This deficiency is due to the excess consumption of vital essence or to fever that impairs vital essence.

A deficiency of *yin* may lead to a relative overabundance of *yang*, accompanied by excessive upward movement, an increase in interior heat, and hyperfunctioning of the deficiency type in the internal organs. *Yin* fails to check *yang*. This failure occurs most commonly in cases of debilitation due to prolonged illness or in the advanced stages of diseases that are accompanied by a high fever.

The resulting symptom-complex is known as "heat due to deficiency of *yin.*" Its symptoms are low fever; erratic fever; feverish sensation in the palms, soles, and the chest; night sweats; dry mouth and throat; and a tongue that is reddened, but with little or no coating. The pulse is feeble and rapid.[12]

IF *YIN* PERISHES. *Yin* is said to perish when there is a severe consumption or loss of vital essence. The most common cause is excessive heat which "scorches" the body's fluids. Other causes include massive hemorrhaging, vomiting, diarrhea, or other chronic conditions that quickly consume vital essence. In comparison with the symptom-complex of *yin* deficiency, this condition is marked by a higher fever. This higher fever is due to profuse sweating or massive vomiting and diarrhea, which lead to severe disorders of water metabolism, including dehydration and loss of blood.

11. In preliminary studies of this symptom-complex, the following pathological changes have been observed: chronic inflammatory changes appear in the diseased organs, especially in advanced stages of disease. Most of the inflamed cells are lymph cells and large uninuclear cells. There is a proliferation of fibrous connective tissue. The physiological functioning of the parenchymal cells is partially damaged. Hypofunctioning, due to the chronic inflammation, is obvious.

In addition, the disturbance of blood circulation produces anemia, ischemia, venous stasis, and edema. These problems may be either systemic or local, and are sometimes followed by a decrease in the metabolic rate of the tissue.

12. The current research on the symptom-complex of heat due to deficient *yin* suggests that the fever may be related to temporary arterial congestion caused by disorders of the autonomic nervous system, especially functional disturbances of the thyroid gland.

The perishing of *yin* is a critical state. The loss of vital essence reduces the concentration of vital energy, since the two are interdependent. Vital energy disperses and "floats" to the body surface. If this situation is not remedied in time, *yang* also perishes soon afterward. The body system collapses, and life is endangered.

IF EXCESSIVE *YIN* HINDERS *YANG*. A preponderance of *yin* produces excessive cold. If the cold is trapped within the body, and *yin* is unable to be released to reach the body surface, *yin* and *yang* then become separated from each other. They repel each other. This condition is described as "excessive *yin* hindering *yang*." The accompanying symptom-complex is known as "true cold and false heat." It has characteristics of excessive internal cold along with symptoms such as fever, a flushed face, thirst, and a long pulse.

Closely related to this condition is the symptom-complex known as "lower true cold and upper false-heat." In this morbid state *yang* is separated from *yin* and floats upward in the body, due to cold in the lower burner. Accordingly, it is known as the "upward floating of *yang*."

IF *YIN* IS IMPAIRED AND IMPEDES THE GENERATION OF *YANG*. The overconsumption of vital essence can lead to insufficient growth of vital energy. The result is a deficiency of *yang*, and, eventually, a deficiency of both vital essence and vital energy.

This condition begins with consumptive pathological changes such as seminal emission, night sweats, and loss of blood. In these cases, vital essence is being so severely consumed that the body fails to produce the material foundation for the growth of vital energy. The result is a symptom-complex of deficiency of *yang*, with spontaneous perspiration, aversion to cold, and diarrhea with watery stools that contain undigested food.

THE FAILURE OF *QI*

In traditional Chinese medicine, *yin, yang, qi,* and blood are seen as materials produced by the *zang-fu* organs. They are distributed to all parts of the body via the channels and vessels to nourish the tissues and organs. In conditions of disease, the primary disorders are those of *yin* and *yang* or of vital essence and energy.

Apart from these, however, are disorders of *qi* and blood, which have the same interdependent relationship as *yin* and *yang*. (See table 6.2.) Blood is the material basis for the generation of *qi;* at the same time, the formation and circulation of blood depends on *qi*. *Qi* plays the leading role in this process. The flow of blood follows the flow of *qi*. A retardation of the flow of *qi* causes stagnation of blood. A prostration of *qi* produces a great loss of blood.

Qi disorders are of four types:

IF *QI* BECOMES DEFICIENT. Deficiency of *qi* occurs primarily in cases of hypofunctioning of the spleen, the kidney, and sometimes the lung. However, it may occur whenever prolonged illness, hypofunctioning, or weakness of the organs and tissues leads to the consumption of vital energy. The following symptoms are characteristic of this condition: lowered body resistance, tendency to perspire, susceptibility to exogenous pathogenic factors, lassitude, and cold limbs due to lack of nourishment. Dizziness and ringing in the ears may also appear since *qi* fails to ascend properly and hence does not sufficiently nourish the sense organs. Because blood is unable to circulate freely in this condition, the vessels become withered, and the pulse tends to be feeble. The retention of water and disturbances in its distribution lead to the formation of phlegm or excessive fluid. Overabundant water and dampness may even cause edema.

IF *QI* BECOMES STAGNANT. *Qi* becomes stagnant when it is obstructed. Obstructions may arise when the *zang-fu* organs fail to function properly or when some other local or systemic disturbance impedes the travel of *qi*. Stagnant *qi* appears most commonly in cases of depression or stagnation of phlegm and dampness.

The retarded flow of *qi* often leads to a stagnation of channel *qi* in particular; blood circulation is also impeded. A sensation of swelling and distension is common, as is localized pain due to blood stasis. Edema and the formation of phlegm are also symptoms of stagnant *qi,* since disturbances in urine secretion and water metabolism hamper the distribution of water and food essence. All of these problems lead, in turn, to a series of disturbances of the *zang-fu* organs, including malfunctioning of the lung, depression of liver *qi,* or stagnation of spleen and stomach *qi.*

IF *QI* SINKS IN THE MIDDLE BURNER. Sinking *qi* is a type of *qi* deficiency. Its trademark is the failure of *qi* to ascend, accompanied by weakness of spleen *qi,* hypofunctioning of the *zang-fu* organs, the downward movement of these organs, and the inability of *qi* to "lift" the tissues.[13] The main causes of sinking *qi* in the middle burner are a poor physique, protracted illness, and a consumption of spleen *qi,* which impedes the upward and downward flow of food essence and waste. Symptoms of sinking *qi* include gastroptosis, nephroptosis, prolapse of the uterus and rectum, distension and heaviness in the abdominal and lumbar regions, lassitude, and a feeble voice. The pulse is thready and forceless.

IF THE FLOW OF *QI* BECOMES ADVERSE. Under certain conditions, the *qi* of the *zang-fu* organs will flow upward when it should not. An abnormal upward flow of the *qi* of the lung, liver, stomach, and Chong Channel is most common. It is usually the result of impaired emotions, excess consumption of cold or raw food, or some obstruction of phlegm or waste.

The abnormal lateral flow of liver *qi* obstructs blood in the upper body, causing dizziness or even coma. The failure of the lung activities of "dispersing and descending" and of the stomach activities of "adjusting and descending" causes lung *qi* and stomach *qi* to flow upward. The result is coughing, asthma, hiccups, nausea, vomiting, a suffocating sensation in the chest, constipation, and the retention of urine.

If the flow of *qi* suddenly becomes adverse, the vessels of the lung and stomach may be impaired; blood will escape from them, leading to the expectoration of blood and hematemesis.

Fright will often cause abnormal flow of liver or kidney *qi* or a condition of cold and dampness along the channels. The *qi* of the Chong Channel will, as a result, flow laterally and upward, causing

---

13. One of the functions of *qi* is to support or "lift" the adjoining tissues of the body; it "holds things in place."

a sensation of gas in the abdomen known in traditional Chinese medicine as "Ben Tun."[14]

THE FAILURE OF BLOOD

There are four types of blood dysfunctions:

IF BLOOD BECOMES DEFICIENT. Blood may fail to nourish the *zang-fu* organs, the vessels, and other parts of the body for several reasons: (1) massive loss of blood without sufficient replenishment; (2) a decreased ability of the spleen and stomach to transform food essence into blood; and (3) internal damage to blood due to protracted illness or intestinal parasites.

In such cases, the lack of nourishment of the body leads to symptoms of weakness, including pallor, pale lips and tongue, dull nails, dizziness and giddiness, continuous violent palpitations, shortness of breath, lassitude, numbness of the hands and feet, stiff joints, dry eyes, and blurred vision.

IF BLOOD BECOMES STAGNANT. Blood circulation may be retarded by the invasion of the blood by pathogenic factors or a blocking of the vessels as a result of exogenous pathogenic factors; by improper treatment of hemorrhaging; by injuries of the vessels due to direct impact; by stagnation of *qi;* and, in women, by retention of the lochia following childbirth. Conditions of stagnant blood are characterized by fixed pains that do not respond to either warm or cold applications. Signs of blood stasis also appear; these include purpura, dark brown eyelids, purplish skin, dark purple lips and tongue or purple spots on the tongue, and dry scaly skin.

Just as stagnant *qi* may retard the circulation of blood, stagnant blood may interfere with the smooth flow of *qi.* Numbness of the limbs, accompanied by local swelling, may then occur.

IF THE BLOOD SYSTEM IS ATTACKED BY HEAT. The symptom-complex of heat in the blood may develop in several ways. Either

14. "Ben Tun" is described as a feeling of masses of gas ascending within the abdomen "like running piggies."

endogenous or exogenous pathogenic heat may invade the blood system. Exogenous cold may also invade the system and be transformed into pathogenic heat.[15] In addition, heat in the blood may develop from prolonged emotional depression that first depresses liver *qi* and eventually results in internal fire. However it develops, heat in the blood damages the blood system by scorching vital essence and by causing the blood to escape from the vessels. Accordingly, symptoms include the typical symptoms of heat, consumption of blood and injury of *yin,* as well as hemorrhaging.

TABLE 6.2. When Disturbances of *Qi* and Blood Interact

Because *qi* and blood interact, the failure of one often brings on disturbances of the other. These compound disturbances produce characteristic sets of symptoms. For example:

Stagnation of qi *and blood stasis.*
Blood circulation depends on *qi.* A retardation of the flow of *qi* causes blood stasis, which leads to pain. Painful masses in the abdomen are characteristic of this condition.

Prostration of qi *after great loss of blood.*
Massive hemorrhaging is often accompanied by simultaneous or subsequent prostration of *qi.* The result is coma, due to deficiency of both blood and *qi* as well as a failure of *yin* and *yang.*

Failure of qi *to control blood.*
Weakness of spleen *qi,* in particular, can lead to abnormal bleeding. The characteristic symptoms are rectal bleeding, blood in the urine, uterine hemorrhaging, and rupturing of blood vessels beneath the skin. These symptoms are accompanied by those of weak spleen *qi* and insufficient spleen *yang.*

Abnormal flow of blood due to abnormal flow of qi.
This condition is traditionally known as the "upward rush of blood after *qi.*" It is characterized by hemorrhaging in the upper portion of the body due to an excessive ascending motion of liver *qi,* upward invasion of the lung by liver fire, or an abnormal upward flow of both lung and stomach *qi.* The symptoms can include hematemesis, spitting up blood, epistaxis, and coma.

Insufficient qi *and blood to nourish the vessels.*
Any derangement of *qi* and blood immediately hinders their ability to nourish the vessels and limbs, creating local deficiencies of *qi* and blood. The characteristic symptom of this condition is numbness of the limbs.

15. The symptom-complex involving the *ying* (nutrient) and *xue* (blood) systems, seen in diseases accompanied by high fever, are the result of this process.

IF HEMORRHAGING OCCURS. Hemorrhaging usually occurs as a result of adverse flow of *qi,* scorching of the vessels by excess fire, or external injury to the vessels. Since blood vessels are present over the entire body, hemorrhaging may occur at any place in the body. The symptoms vary with the location of the hemorrhaging. For example, if the lung is injured, the patient will cough up blood. If the small vessels of the large intestine are injured, rectal bleeding will occur. Blood in the urine appears when the blood vessels of the urinary bladder or urethra are injured. Menorrhagia or uterine hemorrhaging indicate injury to the Chong and Ren Channels. Other typical locations of hemorrhaging are the nose, gums, eyes, skin, and muscles.

Excessive loss of blood leads to a deficiency of both *qi* and blood, as well as a decline in the functioning of the organs and tissues. Sudden loss of large amounts of blood may cause the complete exhaustion of *qi;* death then results from the "divorce of *yin* from *yang."* Disturbances of *qi* and blood interaction are summarized in table 6.2.

FAILURE OF THE ASCENDING AND DESCENDING MOVEMENTS

If there were no entering and exiting of *qi,* there would be no birth, growth, vigor, senility, or death. If there were no ascending and descending, there would be no germination, growth or blossoming; no bearing of fruit nor any harvest. All organisms share in these life processes.

"Treatise on the Six Climatic Factors"
in *Plain Questions*

The interstitial spaces between the skin and flesh are passageways for *qi.* Ascending and descending mean the circulation of the *qi* in the internal organs; entering and exiting mean the exchange of *qi* between interior and exterior. The action of the eyes, ears, nose, tongue, body, and mind is dependent on the smooth flow of *qi.* If the passageways are blocked, their action ceases.

"Essay on the Ascending, Descending,
Entering, and Exiting of *Qi"* in
A Sketch of Medical Study

Qi has four basic patterns of motion: ascending, descending, entering, and exiting. These motions maintain the "harmony of opposites" in the *zang-fu* organs. If these basic patterns of motion are disrupted, the organs, limbs, and orifices of the body will all suffer.

The types of pathological changes that result from failures in the ascending and descending movement of *qi* may be summarized as follows:

- Failure of the lung in dispersing and descending. When lung *qi* does not travel smoothly or when it flows upward instead of downward, discomfort in the chest, coughing, and asthma result.
- Failure of the stomach to send down food content. An abnormal upward movement in the functioning of the stomach causes foul belching, vomiting, and nausea; failure of the stomach to disperse *qi* downward results in loss of appetite.
- Failure of the spleen to send up "clarity" (or food essence). Loose stools or diarrhea are often the result of poor functioning of the spleen in transporting and digesting food.
- Adverse flow of liver *qi* due to hyperfunctioning. An exuberance of liver *yang* causes dizziness and a sensation of distension in the head; the adverse flow of overly exuberant liver *qi* also produces pain in the hypochondriac region and irritability.
- Failure of the kidney to promote inhalation. If the kidney is weak, it is unable to promote inhalation, and the amount of *qi* inhaled is less than the amount exhaled. Shortness of breath and asthmatic breathing result.
- Obstruction of the large intestine. When the downward flow of *qi* in the large intestine fails, constipation results.
- Failure of the descending motion in the urinary bladder. This kind of disturbance results in a weak flow of urine, decreased urination, or even retention of urine.
- Weakness of the spleen and the sinking of *qi*. A deficiency of *qi* in the middle burner (the region of the spleen) means an inability to support the adjoining tissues; the symptoms are prolapse of the rectum and uterus and a sensation of heaviness in the stomach and abdomen.
- Discord between the heart and kidney. When heart fire does not descend to the kidney, and kidney water fails to ascend to the heart, the normal physiological coordination between the heart and kidney breaks down. The resulting symptoms include restlessness, insomnia, palpitation, and poor memory.

Among the various disturbances in the ascending and descending movements of *qi,* disorders of the stomach and spleen are both the most common and the most important.

IN SUMMARY

According to traditional Chinese medicine, two factors are involved in every disease: (1) the pathogenic factor and (2) the antipathogenic *qi* (or the body's resistance). Of these two, antipathogenic *qi* is the more important in determining the course of the disease.

The course of disease can be viewed as a struggle between the pathogenic factor and antipathogenic *qi*. This struggle proceeds according to the laws of *yin* and *yang,* producing two basic types of symptom-complexes: those of excess and those of deficiency. In symptom-complexes of excess the pathogenic factor is preponderant, but antipathogenic *qi* remains strong. In symptom-complexes of deficiency, antipathogenic *qi* is impaired.

In either case, the dynamic equilibrium of the body has been disrupted. The result is: (1) an imbalance of *yin* and *yang;* (2) a derangement of *qi* and blood; or (3) a disturbance in the ascending and descending functions of the organs. The particular characteristics of a disease will depend on which of these disorders occurs.

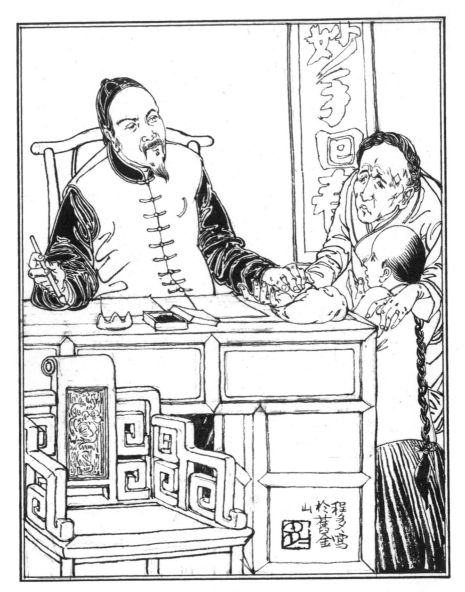

A doctor making a pulse diagnosis of a patient.

CHAPTER SEVEN

Methods of Examination

The patient's complexion and pulse are in accord with the condition of the skin on the forearm. Just as the sound of the drum breaks out in response to the beat of the drumstick, just as the condition of the root is reflected in the leaves of a tree, so the conditions of the complexion, pulse, and muscles of a man cannot be considered as isolated from one another.

"Treatise on the Pathology and Etiology of
Visceral Diseases" in *Miraculous Pivot*

THE GOAL OF all diagnosis in traditional Chinese medicine is to differentiate among symptom-complexes. This is a two-stage process. The first stage is *examination*. The second stage is interpretation: the information gathered by examination is interpreted according to the principles of differentiating symptom-complexes.

The first stage—examination of the patient—is the subject of this chapter. The guiding question in this stage is: What can be known about the patient? More specifically, what can be perceived through the senses?

The *Classic of Internal Medicine* asserts that nothing in the world is beyond knowing. All things, all phenomena in the world are interconnected. Thus, if something cannot be studied directly, its condition may be inferred by investigating those things to which it is related.

In the human body, the *zang-fu* organs are interconnected with each other and with exterior parts of the body via the channels. Any excess or deficiency of *qi* and blood and *yin* and *yang* in the internal organs can be accurately judged by changes in the complexion, the color of the skin, the pulse, and other conditions accessible to the senses. This is the first principle of diagnosis: that "the interior condition can be detected from the exterior."[1]

A second principle that guides diagnosis is *integrity*. According to traditional Chinese medicine, whenever a person is ill, the local condition influences the entire body. Conversely, general pathological changes are often focused on a local area. By observing a local disorder, the practitioner may therefore ascertain the general condition of the body. Furthermore, if an interior disorder cannot be observed directly, the general condition—as reflected in the complexion, pulse, and other observable features of the body—will accurately portray the more interior disorder.

While "nothing in the world is beyond knowing,"[2] inferences based on indirect observations cannot be arbitrary. Therefore, Chinese medicine has evolved a systematic approach to examination. This approach consists of four basic methods: (1) looking; (2) listening; (3) asking; and (4) feeling.[3]

LOOKING: GENERAL AND SPECIFIC INFORMATION FOR DIAGNOSIS

> We may know the condition of someone's internal organs and the place in which the disease occurs by observing the external manifestation.
>   "Treatise on the Original Organs"
>   in *Miraculous Pivot*

Traditional Chinese medicine places a high value on visual inspection as a diagnostic method: since the condition of the interior is

1. "Treatise on the Correspondence between Man and the Universe," in *Plain Questions*. *Danxi's Experimental Therapy* (1280–1358) also states, "If you want to know the internal condition, the external manifestation should be observed, since the internal disorder is bound to be reflected externally." The method of "knowing the interior from the exterior" is similar to the "black box" method of modern cybernetics. This method seeks correlations among the inner components of an object and between the object and its environment in much the same way as traditional Chinese medicine. This method asserts that it is not enough to open or decompose an object when studying it; rather it should be kept intact. Its nature and mode of functioning is inferred through analysis of the external stimuli it receives and the response it makes.

2. This is a fundamental principle expressed throughout the *Classic of Internal Medicine*.

3. These basic methods are sequential, with looking, or observing the patient, as the first step. In Western medical practice, the patient is generally first asked, or interviewed,

reflected on the exterior, examination of the exterior is a key to understanding the nature of any disease. The method of looking and the meaning of what one finds has been systematized over centuries of practice. The traditional practitioner observes the physique, the general expression of the patient, the color of the complexion, the various parts of the head and face, and the tongue. These observations reveal both the general condition of the body—its strength, vitality, and likelihood of recovery—and more specific information about the type of symptom-complex and the afflicted organs.

For example:

The Physique

Body build and patterns of movement indicate the general functioning of the internal organs. The practitioner observes whether the body is weak or strong, obese or emaciated. An obese person is often suffering from a *yang* deficiency as well as profuse phlegm and dampness in the interior. A very thin or emaciated person, on the other hand, frequently suffers from insufficient essence and blood, together with exuberant fire due to a *yin* deficiency.

An abnormal gait or posture may indicate a congenital defect or it may reflect a current disease. For example:

—A lowered head, and a bending back or hanging of the shoulders usually indicate insufficient *qi* of the viscera.
—Motion impairment in the lumbar region and leg joint indicates weakness of the tendons and bones due to lowered functioning of the liver and kidney.
—Convulsions indicate stirring up of wind in the liver.

Characteristic patterns of movement also reveal the general state of a patient. Since "motion is *yang*, while quiescence is *yin*," a tendency to be very active or a preference for moving about points to a *yang* symptom-complex, while a preference for rest suggests a *yin*

followed by other methods of examination. Traditional Chinese medicine places importance on first observing the patient from the moment he is sighted by the practitioner. Since diseases of the interior are reflected on the exterior, by first looking at the patient the practitioner can ascertain his overall condition and preclude any biases that may arise through interview.

symptom-complex. In addition, abnormal body movements such as tremors of the eyelids, mouth, lips, fingers, or toes may be warning signs of endogenous wind arising as a result of (1) extreme heat; (2) malnutrition of vessels due to a deficiency of blood; or (3) hyperfunctioning of liver *yang*.

The Expression

According to traditional Chinese medicine, the expression of a person reveals his or her vitality as well as mental and spiritual state. It is the outward sign of a preponderance or discomfiture of *qi* and blood in the organs. Most important in observing a person's expression are the eyes, which indicate one of three conditions: (1) a vigorous spirit; (2) a lack of vitality; and (3) pseudovitality.

The signs of a vigorous spirit are attentiveness, a sparkle in the eyes, keen response to questions, and clear speech. These signs show that *qi* has not been injured and that the organs are in basically good condition. If the spirit is vigorous, the disease is mild.

Lack of vitality may be inferred when the patient appears spiritless, with dull eyes, a sluggish response, a feeble voice, or possibly some mental disturbance. (Incontinence of urine in serious cases may also signal a lack of vitality.) These signs all indicate that the disease is serious. Vital energy has been damaged, and the prognosis is poor.

Pseudovitality is a false appearance of vitality that occurs in a long, serious disease when the patient's vital energy is severely depleted. The practitioner may suspect pseudovitality when

—The patient has been apathetic and breathing feebly, but suddenly becomes excessively talkative;
—The patient suddenly switches from very low spirits to very high spirits; or
—The patient's face has been pale but suddenly becomes flushed.

Such abrupt changes in expression do not follow the normal course of disease and recovery. They are critical signs of the imminent divorce of *yin* from *yang* (due to excessive *yang* hindering *yin* or the failure of *yin* to hold *yang*). They are thus usually known as "the last radiance of the setting sun" or the "reglowing of a candle that is about to burn out." They demand special attention since they signal a serious deterioration.

Color of the Complexion

Abnormal color and lusterless skin are signs of illness. In cases of mild disease, the skin will retain its normal color and luster, indicating that *qi* and blood are still adequate. If the complexion is dull and shriveled, however, the condition is serious; such a complexion indicates that vital energy has been damaged and that the prognosis is poor.

In addition to establishing the general condition of the body, the complexion can indicate specific disorders. According to traditional Chinese medicine, there are five basic colors—green, yellow, red, white, and black—that correspond to the condition of the organs and to various pathogenic factors. For example:

—A green complexion often refers to an obstruction of the vessels due to coagulation of pathogenic cold and *qi* stagnation; symptom-complexes of cold, pains, and stagnant blood (or perhaps infantile convulsions) are likely.

—Yellow skin may imply a weakened spleen with excess dampness and a symptom-complex of deficiency or dampness in the spleen.

—A red complexion suggests excessive flow of blood in the vessels due to exuberant heat; the symptom-complex is probably one of heat. If the face is flushed, a fever due to exogenous affection or a heat symptom-complex is likely. Flushed cheeks indicate a symptom-complex of *yin* deficiency due to exuberant *yang* in the internal organs.

—A very white complexion suggests that the blood and *qi* are in poor condition because of deficiency of *yang* and decrease of *qi*, and that there is insufficient blood in the vessels because of consumption of *qi* or loss of blood; both of these conditions will produce a pallid countenance, indicating a deficiency symptom-complex of cold or hemorrhaging.

—Black in the complexion indicates weakened kidneys and an excess of cold and water transformed from accumulation of endogenous dampness. The symptom-complex is most likely one of phlegm, stagnant blood, *yang* deficiency, and a decline in fire; these conditions produce abundant dampness and cold in the interior and a failure in the nourishing and warming of blood. Ultimately, they may lead to contraction of the vessels and failure of the blood to flow smoothly. This is the cause of dark shadows in the face.

Secretions and Excretions of the Body

The secretions of the human body include nasal discharge, tears, sputum, saliva, and vaginal discharge. Feces and urine are classified as excretions. The color, quantity, and texture of both secretions and excretions indicate the condition of the body. For example:

—If secretions or excretions are white, dilute, and clear, they indicate a symptom-complex of cold.
—If secretions or excretions are yellow, thick, and sticky, they suggest a symptom-complex of heat.
—Large amounts of secretions and excretions indicate abundant dampness or a deficiency symptom-complex of cold.
—Scanty secretions and excretions indicate consumption and lack of body fluid.

Blood sometimes appears in the secretions and excretions of the body. In these cases, there is a possibility that the vessels have been damaged by heat. More specifically:

—Bloody sputum or coughing up blood indicates injury to the vessels of the lung. Coughing up blood together with pus usually indicates a pulmonary abscess.
—Bloody stools, accompanied by pus, may indicate a downward pouring of damp-heat, which injures the vessels of the intestines; the decaying tissues of the intestines turn to pus.
—Blood in the urine indicates injury to the vessels of the urinary bladder and urethra due to a pouring down of damp heat.

The Head and Face

Through all of the 12 principal channels and 360 collateral channels, blood and *qi* travel up to the face and through the orifices.

"Treatise on the Pathology and Etiology of
Visceral Diseases" in *Miraculous Pivot*

The hair, eyes, ears, nose, lips, teeth, throat, and facial skin are all closely linked to the internal organs by the channels. Their external form, color, and secretions thus mirror the state of these organs as well as the condition of *qi* and blood. For example,

—In children, a head that appears too large or too small—when accompanied by mental retardation—often suggests a deficiency of kidney essence.

—Sparse hair, premature loss of hair, or dry and withered hair may be related to a deficiency of essence and blood.

—A yellowish color in the whites of the eyes often indicates jaundice.

—Red and swollen upper eyelids may indicate an injury to the Liver Channel by wind-heat.

—Shriveled and blackened ears may indicate a consumption of kidney essence.

—An inflammation of the middle ear or accumulation of excessive earwax may indicate dampness and heat in the liver and gallbladder.

—A running nose with a watery discharge indicates an attack by exogenous wind-cold.

—A running nose with a thick discharge indicates an attack by wind-heat.

—Prolonged thick, foul nasal discharge indicates an inflammation of the sinuses, usually caused by heat which has accumulated in the Gallbladder Channel due to exogenous pathogens.

—Ulcers in the mouth or on the lips commonly indicate an abnormal upward flow of accumulated heat in the spleen and stomach.

—Deviations of the mouth and eyes (e.g., Bell's palsy) occur when the channel system is attacked by pathogenic wind.

—Trembling in newborns or persistent tics may indicate a stirring of wind in the liver.

—Dryness of the gums can indicate a serious injury to body fluid caused by exuberant heat in the stomach.

—Red, swollen, and bleeding gums indicate an injury to the vessels due to the upward flaming of stomach heat.

—A red, sore, and swollen or ulcerous throat, covered with yellow or white spots, usually indicates the accumulation of exuberant heat in the lungs and stomach.

—Puffy skin that feels like soft mud when pressed suggests a disturbance in metabolism of water or dampness.

The Tongue

Traditional Chinese medicine places much emphasis on the inspection of the tongue as a method of diagnosis. The tongue is a mirror of the heart as well as the outward or external reflection of the spleen and stomach. It is connected both directly and indirectly with several *zang-fu* organs via the channels. For instance, the Heart Channel communicates with the base of the tongue. The Spleen Channel joins the base of the tongue and then spreads out over its lower surface. The Kidney Channel divides and travels along the two sides of the base of the tongue. The Liver Channel as well as the branches of the Urinary Bladder Channel and the Heart Channel also join the base of the tongue. Accordingly, the tongue provides a complex picture of the essence and *qi* of the internal organs.

Modern medicine recognizes three types of papillae, or projections, on the tongue: filiform, fungiform, and circumvallate. Two of these— the fungiform and filiform—have been important in Chinese medical diagnosis since early times. The fungiform papillae are known as "red granules"; the filiform are called "soft thorns" by the ancient Chinese medical scholars. They write:

> The red granules, which are as fine as millet and are located on the tip of the tongue, are projections of the heart *qi* and are associated with genuine fire of the vital gate. The whitish soft thorns that look like hair on the surface of the tongue are produced by lung *qi* and are also associated with genuine fire of the vital gate.
>
> *A Synopsis of Diagnostic Observations
> of Appearance and Color*

The tongue muscles are red due to the numerous blood vessels that flow into them and into the lower layer of the mucous membrane. However, the normal, healthy tongue does not appear bright red. It is coated by a white translucent mucous with a cornified layer; this coating gives the tongue a light red color. It is formed by the filiform papillae or soft thorns. Each of these are partially cornified at their ends, forming a kind of tree structure. The spaces between these soft pricks are filled with cornified tissue that has been shed, as well as saliva, germs, broken bits of food, and leukocytes (blood cells) that have been secreted. All of these combine to form the normal thin whitish coating.

A normal, healthy tongue, then, is light red in color; it moves freely; and it is covered by a thin white coating with evenly spread granules. The surface is neither dry nor overly moist.

For diagnostic purposes, the tongue can be divided into four portions, which correspond to the organs as follows:

—The tip corresponds to the heart and lung.
—The middle corresponds to the spleen and stomach.
—The root corresponds to the kidney.
—The edges correspond to the liver and gallbladder.[4]

In addition, the tongue should be inspected for its general color, its shape, and the type of coating.

For example, the general color of the tongue reveals the strength of antipathogenic *qi* and the body's vitality. It also indicates whether the symptom-complex is one of deficiency or excess. More specifically:

—A pale tongue indicates symptom-complexes of deficiency and cold, caused by deficiency of *yang qi* and insufficiency of blood and *qi*.[5]
—A reddened tongue indicates a symptom-complex of interior heat caused by excess of *qi* and blood in the vessels. It may be due either to excess or to *yin* deficiency. A dry reddened tongue indicates endogenous heat due to *yin* deficiency, while a reddened tongue with coating indicates excess heat.[6]
—A deep red tongue is a sign of severe endogenous heat. Usually it represents a deterioration from the condition of a reddened tongue. It appears in patients with exuberant heat in the *ying* and *xue* systems[7] or in those suffering from consumption of fluid.[8]

4. While these relationships have proved useful in diagnosis, the mechanism of their relationship remains to be explored.

5. From a Western point of view, it might be assumed that a pale tongue usually occurs when there is a contraction in the capillaries and a decrease in the blood volume or circulatory flow. It is a possible sign of anemia, hypoproteinemia, functional disorders of the digestive system, a low basal rate of metabolism, or inadequate glandular secretions.

6. A reddened tongue may be related to problems of dilation and contraction of the capillaries; an increase in metabolism; an increase in the concentration of blood due to high fever; dehydration; and lack of vitamin B. It is typical in cases of acute infectious diseases, burns, hyperthyroidism, malignant tumors, acute hepatitis, cirrhosis, hepatic coma, tuberculosis, sunstroke, and diabetes.

7. For a definition of the *ying* and *xue* systems, see note 16, chapter 1.

8. A deep red tongue may reflect: (1) abnormal dilation and constriction of numerous capillaries together with an increased blood volume; or (2) a concentration or agglutination

—A blue or purple tongue indicates stagnation of blood. A purple
tongue with deep red coloration indicates inadequate fluid; it suggests that an exuberant pathogenic heat has led to consumption of
fluid or an irregular flow of *qi* and blood. A pale purple or moist
blue-purple tongue indicates a blockage of vessels due to preponderant endogenous cold. Purple spots on the tongue also suggest
a stagnation of blood. A purple tongue occurs commonly in cases
of liver or gallbladder trouble or in heart diseases.[9] A blue-purple
tongue occurs most commonly in cases of severe heart failure or
respiratory failure. A dry purple tongue is typically associated
with infectious diseases accompanied by a high fever.[10]

Chinese medicine also stresses the shape and surface condition of
the tongue as important diagnostic information:

—A flabby pale tongue may indicate a failure in the transformation
of body fluids and a retention of phlegm and dampness due to a
deficiency of spleen and kidney *yang*.[11]
—A swollen, deep red tongue indicates exuberant heat in the heart
and spleen. It may also be seen in local infections of the tongue.
—A swollen, dark blue-purple tongue usually indicates poisoning.
—A thin, shrunken tongue indicates consumption and deficiency of
yin.[12]
—A cracked tongue indicates consumption of vital essence, which
fails to nourish the tongue's surface.[13]

of blood due to dehydration. It typically occurs in cases where there is a disturbance in
water metabolism due to dehydration in the late stages of a febrile disease or in serious liver
conditions, in advanced stages of cancer, and in coma cases.

9. The purple tongue may be related to reduced hemoglobin as a result of blood stagnation in the veins or lack of oxygen. In addition, a purple tongue can be a sign of ery-
throcytosis, alcoholism, cor pulmonale, an increase of cold causing agglutination of the
blood cells, or cancer.

10. In this case, circulatory disturbances may retard the blood flow, lower the saturation
of blood oxygen, produce blood stagnation, and mechanically alter the coagulation of blood.

11. Preliminary studies in China suggest that the flabby pale tongue may be related to
chronic digestive problems, decreases in serum albumin (blood protein), enlargement of the
spine cells, excessive growth of connective tissues, edema of the tongue, decreased functioning of the endocrine system, and disturbances in water metabolism. It is common in cases
of myxedema, acromegaly, anemia, chronic nephritis, or nephrosis.

12. The thin, shrunken tongue appears to occur in cases of malnutrition, tuberculosis,
anemia, advanced tumors, and pellagra.

13. In Western terms, this tongue condition may be related to atrophy of the mucous
membrane or fusion of the papillae of the tongue. It occurs in cases of dehydration due to
high fever, malnutrition, a deficiency of riboflavin, and anemia.

—A tongue with teeth imprints along the outer edge indicates a deficiency symptom-complex of the spleen. If the tongue is also weakened, the weakened spleen has probably produced a condition of preponderant cold and dampness.[14]

—A thorny tongue is due to exuberant pathogenic heat. The more exuberant the heat is, the more "thorns" will appear on the tongue.[15]

—A rigid tongue may result from exogenous affection by heat. In this case, invasion of the pericardium by heat produces accumulation of phlegm and eventually an obstruction in the body's interior. A rigid tongue may also result from undernourishment of the vessels due to impaired body fluids in cases of high fever. If it accompanies other internal disorders, it is often a sign of impending stroke.

—A weak tongue that is flaccid in appearance indicates a consumption of *yin* fluid and a consequent failure to nourish the tendons due to extreme deficiency of *qi* and blood.

—A trembling tongue indicates a deficiency of both *qi* and blood or a stirring of endogenous wind due to deficiency.

—A tendency to stick out the tongue or to play with it suggests excess heat in the spleen.

—A deviated tongue indicates the imminent possibility of stroke.

—A short contracted tongue is a sign of critical disease and should be taken into special consideration.

Finally, the tongue coating reveals the condition of the body. Traditional Chinese medicine states that the tongue coating is produced by the "upward steaming" of stomach *qi:*

> The tongue coating is created by the upward steaming and fuming of stomach *qi,* which is the source of nourishment for the five *zang* organs. The condition of the tongue coating thus tells us the condition of the five *zang* organs. In this way, observation of the tongue coating assists diagnosis.
>
> *A Synopsis of Diagnostic Observation*
> *of Appearance and Color*

14. Such a tongue condition may be directly related to abnormal enlargement of the tongue or a lack of muscular tension in the tongue.

15. The direct cause of this condition appears to be atrophy or cornification and shedding of the filiform papillae and proliferation or excessive growth of the fungiform papillae. This tongue condition occurs commonly in serious illnesses such as pneumonia, infectious encephalitis, scarlet fever, or other cases of high fever.

The tongue coating of a healthy person is thin and whitish, moderately moist, and neither smooth nor dry. When a person is ill, the tongue coating may take on either an abnormal color or an abnormal texture. Abnormalities of color may be interpreted as follows:

—A white coating indicates either an exogenous symptom-complex or one of cold. While a thin white coating is normal, a markedly white coating may sometimes be a sign of exogenous pathogenic wind-cold. A thin white coating with a reddened tongue tip indicates exogenous pathogenic wind-heat. A white but very smooth coating suggests cold-dampness or phlegm in the interior of the body. A white sticky coating indicates phlegm or spleen trouble caused by pathogenic dampness. A combination of exogenous pathogenic factors and exuberant heat in the interior produces a powderlike white coating. [16]

—A yellow coating indicates a symptom-complex of heat in the interior. When exogenous pathogens transform into heat after invading the interior of the body, the tongue coating turns from white to yellow. The deeper yellow the coating, the more severe the interior heat is. A dry yellow coating indicates that the body fluid has been damaged by exuberant heat. A thick, yellow, thorny coating indicates the accumulation of excessive heat, while a yellow, sticky coating indicates both excessive dampness and heat. [17]

—A grey or black tongue indicates an interior symptom-complex—either of extreme heat or abundant cold. A dry black coating indicates a symptom-complex of excess heat in the interior while a smooth greyish-black coating suggests a symptom-complex of excess cold due to a *yang* deficiency. A black coating usually develops out of a grey coating. A black coating occurs in cases such as

16. Modern medicine suggests that the growth of papillae on the tongue, along with an accumulation of a white coating, is due primarily to dyspepsia. Dyspepsia tends to reduce the food intake and decrease salivary secretions, both of which reduce the mechanical friction and self-cleaning action of the tongue; they also may produce nutritional disturbances and abnormal metabolism of the surface (epithelial) cells.

17. Modern studies link the yellow coating to: (1) disorders of the digestive system caused by infections and fever due to inflammation; (2) metabolic disturbances due to functional disorders of the autonomic nervous system; (3) local metabolic disturbances in the cells of the tongue; and (4) abnormal secretion of the oral glands. It is believed that a yellow coating appears when there is a decrease in salivary secretion and self-cleansing action as the result of the proliferation and cornification of filiform papillae, together with local inflammatory secretions of the tongue and the effects of chromogenic bacteria.

dehydration due to high fever, digestive disorders, chronic inflammation, and poisoning.[18]

Abnormalities of the texture of the tongue coating indicate the strength of the pathogen, the likely path of the disease, the relative strength of the pathogenic and antipathogenic factors, changes in the body fluid, and the state of stomach *qi*. For example:

—A thin coating indicates a mild condition in which the pathogenic factor is acting primarily in the exterior layer of the body.
—A thick coating indicates a severe condition in which the pathogenic factor has penetrated the interior of the body. It may also appear when there is an accumulation of undigested food, phlegm, or dampness. In general, thickening of the coating indicates an advance of the disease; when the coating becomes thinner, the disease is alleviated, and the pathogenic factors are eliminated.
—If a moist coating turns dry, the body fluid has been damaged, usually by exuberant heat or the consumption of fluid. If a dry coating turns moist, the pathogenic heat has subsided, and the fluid has been replenished.
—A sticky coating is a layer of turbid, slimy fur on the tongue. It is usually due to the inhibition of *yang qi* by pathogenic factors of *yin* nature, such as phlegmatic dampness or undigested food. It is common in infectious diseases caused by dampness or in cases of illness due to accumulation of phlegm.
—A curd-like coating is a thick, soft, flabby coating with large granules that resemble crushed bean curd. It is formed by the upward steaming of turbid, stale *qi* from the stomach due to exuberant heat. It is common in cases of dyspepsia or retention of phlegm.
—A peeled coating occurs when the coating is partially or completely peeled, leaving behind a permanently bare, smooth surface. It indicates that vital energy and vital essence of the stomach have been damaged or that vital essence of the stomach has been completely exhausted.
—A solid coating is one that is difficult to remove. It indicates, in

18. A black coating may be linked to functional disorders of the central nervous system and multiplication of fungi and chomogenic bacteria. It appears to be the result of brownish-black cornified cells that are produced by the excessive proliferation of black fungi.

particular, the existence of stomach *qi* and appears most commonly in cases of an excess symptom-complex of heat.
—A soft coating that is easy to remove indicates an exhaustion of
stomach *qi* and is usually seen in symptom-complexes of cold and
deficiency.

LISTENING: CLUES TO THE BODY'S CONDITION

The way in which people speak—with an energetic or feeble voice
or in high- or low-pitched tones—provides specific clues about their
state of health or illness. So do the sounds of their breathing and
digestion. These clues point to various symptom-complexes and help
determine the state of *qi* flow in the *zang-fu* organs.

For example, regarding the speaking voice:

—Speaking energetically in high-pitched tones may indicate an excess symptom-complex of heat.
—Speaking feebly in a low-pitched voice often indicates a deficiency
symptom-complex of cold.
—Verbosity, in general, is a sign of heart trouble.

The sounds of breathing are also informative. For example:

—Feeble breathing may indicate a deficiency of *qi* in the lung and
stomach.
—Forceful breathing suggests an excess symptom-complex of heat in
which pathogenic heat blocks the *qi* passageways.
—Loud, coarse breathing and a sonorous voice indicate excess symptom-complexes, usually due to the unsmooth flow of *qi* and to
pathogenic factors in the lung.
—Low feeble panting and intermittent breathing in which the patient exhales more than he or she inhales may be due to the failure of the kidney to help maintain normal inspiration when there
is a deficiency of *qi* in the lung and kidney.
—Faint breathing, together with shortness of breath, indicates a
general deficiency of *qi*.
—A smothering feeling in the chest that is relieved by deep sighing
usually indicates a stagnation of *qi* due to depression of the liver.

Coughing is a special case of breathing. It is the result of an adverse flow of *qi* due to failure in the dispersing and descending functions of the lung. As a rule:

—Coughing with a coarse voice indicates a symptom-complex of excess.
—Coughing with a low, weak voice indicates a symptom-complex of deficiency.
—A dry cough with scanty or thick, sticky sputum indicates either an invasion of the lung by pathogenic dryness or dryness of the lung due to *yin* deficiency.

Hiccupping and belching are disorders caused by the abnormal upward flow of stomach *qi*. Their sounds and odors [19] are indicative of symptom-complexes. For example:

—Hiccups that are loud, short, and forceful may indicate excess heat.
—Belching sounds that are low, long, and feeble usually indicate a deficiency symptom-complex of cold.
—Belching accompanied by a fetid and acid odor indicates dyspesia in which undigested food is retained in the stomach.
—Repeated belching with no odor indicates either a disharmony of the liver and stomach or a backward flow of *qi* due to deficiency of stomach *qi*.

ASKING: WHAT THE PATIENT CAN REVEAL

According to Zhang Jingyue, a physician of the Ming Dynasty (1368–1644), inquiry is "the key to diagnosis and the crux of clinical work."

Like Western medical practitioners, traditional Chinese practitioners interview the patient and his or her family to determine the patient's major complaints, the development and duration of the ill-

19. The method of listening is also known as "auscultation." "Olfaction," or using odors as a means of diagnosis, is usually included in this method, perhaps because of its close connection with the breath. Additional diagnostic information can be found in the odors of various secretions and excretions.

ness, the past history, lifestyle and diet, and family history. Chinese medicine places particular emphasis on understanding the patient's chief complaint in the context of more general information. This general information is gathered according to a formula developed over centuries of practice and known today as "The Ten Questions." The topics of "The Ten Questions" are:

Chills and Fever

The first task of the inquiry is to determine the severity and frequency of fever and chills. Fever and chills are one of the key indicators used to determine the location of the illness—whether it is interior or exterior. For example:

—A fever that starts abruptly and is accompanied by chills usually indicates an exterior symptom-complex caused by an exogenous pathogenic factor. If the fever is slight, but the chills are extreme, the symptom-complex is one of cold in the exterior. High fever with slight chills usually denotes a symptom-complex of heat in the exterior.
—Alternating chills and fever suggest a symptom-complex that is half interior and half exterior.
—A high fever without chills indicates a symptom-complex of heat in the interior.
—A prolonged disease with erratic fever (particularly with low fever in the afternoon) usually suggests a symptom-complex of *yin* deficiency.
—A prolonged disease characterized by an intolerance of cold and preference for warmth with no accompanying fever usually indicates a symptom-complex of *yang* deficiency.

Perspiration

The purpose of asking about perspiration is to determine whether or not sweating is occurring, when it is occurring, and how much it is occurring. Answers to these questions are usually evaluated after the practitioner has determined whether the symptom-complex is an interior or exterior symptom-complex. For example:

—In an exterior symptom-complex, the absence of sweat may indicate an excess condition caused by pathogenic wind-cold.

—In an exterior symptom-complex, the presence of sweat usually
indicates a deficiency condition caused by pathogenic wind or
pathogenic wind-heat.

—In an interior symptom-complex, spontaneous sweating—that is,
breaking out in a sweat during the day—typically indicates a
symptom-complex of *yang* deficiency.

—In an interior symptom-complex, night sweats usually indicates a
symptom-complex of *yin* deficiency.

—Profuse sweating, cold sweating, or sticky and greasy sweat is a
critical sign of exhaustion of *yang qi*.

—Sweating that occurs only on the head is often caused by pathogenic heat in the upper burner or by the "steaming of accumulated dampness" in the middle burner.

—Sweating that occurs on the forehead of aged persons with asthma
may indicate a symptom-complex of deficiency.

—Sweating on one side of the body but not the other results from
the blockage of vessels by wind-phlegm or wind-dampness and is
usually seen in cases of stroke or arthralgia due to wind-dampness.

Pain in the Head, Trunk, and Limbs

Questions about pain focus on its onset, character, and duration.
Chinese medicine distinguishes among several types of pain. For example:

—*Distending* pain is usually due to stagnation of *qi*.

—*Stabbing* pain is usually due to stagnation of blood.

—*Gaseous* pain results from an obstruction of the flow of *qi* due to
pathogenic factors of excess.

—*Burning* pain usually indicates pathogenic fire or a preponderance
of *yang* heat due to *yin* deficiency.

—Pain *accompanied by a sensation of cold* is usually due to obstruction
of the channels by pathogenic cold.

—*Dull* pain often points to an irregular flow of both *qi* and blood.

When asking specifically about pain in the head, trunk, and limbs,
the Chinese practitioner makes the following kinds of evaluations:

—Long-term headaches consisting of many short episodes of pain may be due to exogenous pathogenic wind-cold; they are often accompanied by other indicators of an exterior symptom-complex.

—Intermittent headaches, each of long duration, suggest endogenous pathogenic factors.

—Distending pain in the head, accompanied by dizziness, a flushed face, and red eyes suggests exuberant *yang* in the liver.

—Headache accompanied by dizziness, ringing in the ears, and pain in the lumbar region may indicate a deficiency symptom-complex of the kidney.

—Pain in the lower back may be related to a deficiency symptom-complex of the kidney.

—A migrating pain in the costal region suggests a depression of the liver and the stagnation of *qi*.

—Numbness in the limbs or scalp of obese people is due to obstruction of the collateral channels by damp-phlegm and is often a sign of imminent stroke. If this symptom is present in emaciated people, it is due to malnutrition of the vessels resulting from a deficiency of *qi* and blood.

Sensations in the Chest and Abdomen

In addition to pain, patients may experience a variety of sensations in the chest and abdomen. Some of these pains and sensations may be interpreted as follows:

—A fixed pain in the chest with frequent relapse may denote stagnation of both blood and *qi*.

—Chest pain, accompanied by fever, a suffocating sensation in the chest, and a bitter taste in the mouth may indicate dampness and heat in the liver and gallbladder.

—Distending pain in the chest often suggests heart or lung trouble.

—Pain and a sensation of suffocation in the chest, accompanied by fever and cough, may be due to a symptom-complex of excess heat in the lung.

—A suffocating sensation in the chest and shortness of breath with feeble coughing suggests a weakness of lung *qi*.

—Constricting pain over the sternum may indicate the stagnation of blood in the heart.

—Pain in the stomach is often due to invasion of the stomach by pathogenic cold, the retention of undigested food in the stomach, or a disturbance of the stomach due to perverted flow of liver *qi*.

—When abdominal pain is present, disorders of the stomach, intestines, urinary bladder, and uterus should be considered.

—Acute pain in the right lateral region of the lower abdomen, accompanied by fever and nausea, may indicate an abdominal abscess (e.g., appendicitis).

—Abdominal pain, accompanied by lumps, indicates stagnation of blood.

Defecation and Urination

Frequency and color are the principal characteristics to be judged in inquiries about defecation and urination. For example:

—Constipation in the elderly, in women who have just given birth, and in those suffering from a prolonged illness may denote a deficiency of *qi* or inadequate body fluid.

—Diarrhea in which stools are yellowish brown, accompanied by a burning sensation in the anus and an urgent need to urinate or defecate, suggests a symptom-complex of damp-heat.

—Dry stools may indicate a symptom-complex of excess heat.

—Watery, cold stools containing undigested food indicate a deficiency symptom-complex of cold.

—Diarrhea before daybreak suggests a deficiency of kidney *yang*.

—A scanty amount of deep yellow urine may result from a symptom-complex of excess heat.

—Clear, profuse urine may result from a deficiency symptom-complex of cold.

—Frequent urination, bed-wetting, and incontinence may be due to a deficiency of *qi*.

—Frequent but difficult urination, accompanied by a burning sensation or stabbing pain may be due to the accumulation of damp heat.

Appetite

A poor appetite, accompanied by loose stools or a sensation of fullness in the stomach and abdomen, generally points to weakness of the spleen and stomach. For example:

—Foul belching, acidic regurgitation, and an aversion to the smell of food after eating all suggest an abnormal retention of food.

—A poor appetite, accompanied by a sticky sensation in the mouth and a greasy tongue coating, may result from a disturbance in the spleen and stomach due to dampness.

—If the above condition is relieved after eating, it may be a deficiency symptom-complex. If the condition continues or worsens after eating, it may be symptom-complex of excess.

—A preference for cold food may imply a symptom-complex of heat.

—A preference for hot food may indicate a symptom-complex of cold.

—A bitter taste in the mouth indicates the presence of fire in the liver and gallbladder.

—A sweet taste in the mouth suggests a condition of damp-heat in the spleen.

—The absence of taste sensations suggests either an internal obstruction by pathogenic dampness or a deficiency symptom-complex of cold.

Thirst

A person's preferences for beverages often reveal the body's condition. For example:

—Thirst, accompanied by the desire for beverages, is seen frequently in a symptom-complex of interior heat.

—An absence of thirst or thirst without the desire for beverages appears most frequently in symptom-complexes of cold or severe dampness.

Hearing

The purpose of inquiry about hearing is to determine if there are symptoms of tinnitus, deafness, ear pain, hypoacusis (reduction in ability to perceive sound). For example:

—A serious ear ringing that starts suddenly indicates an excess condition due to flaring up of fire and wind in the Gallbladder Channel.

—A mild ear ringing indicates a deficiency condition due to insufficient vital essence of the liver and kidney.

—Sudden deafness usually suggests a symptom-complex of excess caused by upward attack of pathogenic wind-heat or endogenous heat of the liver and gallbladder, or caused by pathogenic damp-heat that interferes with the mind.

—Deafness developed gradually after prolonged illness or accompanied by ear ringing usually suggests a condition of deficiency caused by a weakened kidney or insufficient *qi* and blood.

—Ear pains mostly denote an upward attack of wind-heat or suppuration in the ears.

—Hypoacusis usually implies dysfunction of the kidney caused by insufficiency of vital essence and energy.

Previous History of Disease

Information about the previous history of disease includes both the patient's and the family's, which provides valuable ground for making a correct diagnosis of the present illness.

Asking about previous disease of the patient, its process of treatment, and condition of relapse may help the practitioner know the condition of the patient's body resistance and the relationship between previous and present illnesses. For instance, if the patient has a previous history of pulmonary tuberculosis, deficiency of vital essence should be considered; if the patient has been afflicted with heart disease or nephritis, deficiency of *qi* should be considered.

The practitioner should also inquire about the family history of disease, especially some communicable or hereditary diseases, such as pulmonary tuberculosis, leprosy, syphilis, and congenital diseases.

Onset and Development of the Present Illness.

This inquiry denotes questioning the entire process of the disease prior to the first visit, including the time, form, and characteristics of the onset, as well as the inducing cause. For example, onset occurring in winter often refers to exogenous affection by pathogenic cold; onset occurring in summer often refers to affection by pathogenic heat or heat stroke; a sudden and rapid advance usually suggests a symptom-complex of excess and heat; while a gradual onset

and slow advance usually denotes a symptom-complex of deficiency
and cold.

Special Questions for Women and Children

In addition to these basic ten areas of inquiry, the Chinese practitioner has special questions for women and children.

With women patients, the practitioner typically asks about menstruation and vaginal discharge. For example:

—A shortened menstrual cycle, with a flow that is excessive in
  amount and deep red in color, may indicate a symptom-complex
  of heat and excess.
—A prolonged cycle with a scanty, light-colored discharge indicates
  a symptom-complex of cold and deficiency.
—Premenstrual distending pain in the abdomen, together with a
  purplish menstrual discharge that has clots, often indicates stagnation of *qi* and blood.
—Postmenstrual abdominal pain that can be relieved by applying
  pressure often indicates a symptom-complex of blood deficiency.
—A whitish, watery vaginal discharge may indicate a symptom-
  complex of cold.
—A thick, yellow vaginal discharge with an offensive odor suggests
  a symptom-complex of damp-heat.
—A continuous white vaginal discharge, or one that resembles
  eggwhites and is accompanied by pain in the lumbar region may
  indicate a deficiency symptom-complex of the kidney.

The practitioner should also ask about the history of any pregnan-
cies. If dizziness, numbness, or even tics of the limbs occur during
the middle or late stages of pregnancy, the possibility of eclampsia
(a form of toxemia) should be considered. A heavy pain in the abdomen, with vaginal bleeding and soreness and pain in the lumbar
region, may indicate impending miscarriage. After childbirth, a constant vaginal discharge, accompanied by abdominal pain, often indicates a failure to discharge stagnant blood.

When treating children, the practitioner should inquire about the
mother's condition before giving birth, any history of measles, chicken
pox, high fever, convulsions, contact with contagious diseases, in-

noculations, the circumstances surrounding their weaning, and their developmental progress in activities such as walking and talking. Inquiry about possible causes of present illness, such as whether the child has a cold, has suffered a fright, or has overeaten are also useful in diagnosing certain diseases. For example:

—Preference for huddling up in a warm place or for being cuddled may indicate a symptom-complex of cold.
—Heat felt inside the mouth suggests a symptom-complex of heat.
—Fever with a hot sensation in the head and trunk with cold limbs suggests exogenous affection by pathogenic wind-cold.
—Fever with hot sensation in the head and coma is a sign of convulsion.
—Fever with rigidity of the neck indicates endogenous wind stirred up by extreme heat or infantile convulsions.

FEELING: THE PULSE AS A GRAPH
OF THE BODY'S CONDITION

Feeling—or palpation—is the fourth method of examining a patient in traditional Chinese medicine. The practitioner feels the limbs and trunk to determine such conditions as the rigidity or suppleness of the chest and abdomen; an abnormal temperature of the hands or feet; the existence of lumps or masses in the abdomen; or the presence of edema. Most important, however, is the pulse. To understand the significance of the pulse in traditional Chinese medicine, one must return to the premise that the body is an organic whole, that the circulation of *qi* and blood through the channels and vessels is closely related to the condition of the internal organs. Not only does the circulation of *qi* and blood convey food essence to the organs, limbs, bones, and various body tissues, but it also regulates the functional harmony of the *zang-fu* organs. Similarly, any pathological condition of the *zang-fu* organs, the *qi* and blood, or the balance of *yin* and *yang* is bound to be reflected in the vessels. Thus, the pulse not only reveals the condition of the heart, but also the general functioning of the body, including its resistance and the likely path of disease.

Traditional Chinese medicine has thus evolved a well-defined method

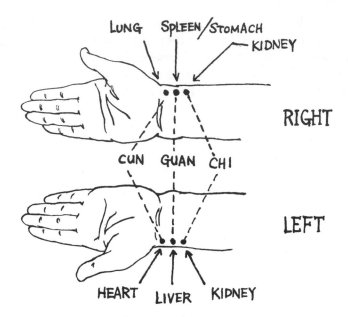

FIGURE 7.1. Pulse Positions and Corresponding Organs

for taking the pulse and interpreting the results. The *Classic of Internal Medicine* instructs the practitioner to feel the pulse on the head, hands, and feet.[20] Today, however, there is one primary location for pulse-taking. This is the *cun kou,* or the area next to the crease in the wrist where the radial artery throbs.[21]

The area known as the *cun kou* is divided into three regions (see figure 7.1). The *guan* is the region opposite the styloid process of the radius. Between the *guan* and the wrist joint is the *cun.* On the other side is the *chi.* Each of these regions corresponds to one of the internal organs. On the right hand, the *cun, guan,* and *chi* reflect the condition of the lung, spleen/stomach, and kidney (vital gate), respectively. On the left hand, the *cun, gaun* and *chi* correspond to the heart, liver, and kidney, respectively.

20. See "An Overall Pulse-Taking Method" in *Plain Questions.* The *Treatise on Cold-Induced Diseases,* by Zhang Zhongjing also suggests three locations for pulse taking: the *ren ying* (the arteria carotis communis), the *cun kou* (the radial artery at the wrist), and the *fu yang* (the arteria dorsalis pedis).

21. Under certain conditions, such as the critical stage of an illness, when the *cun kou* pulse is impalpable, the pulse may be taken at the *ren ying, fu yang,* or *tai xi,* the latter of which lie on the posterior tibial artery.

The *cun kou* is a significant location for pulse taking for several reasons. First, it is the point that reflects the condition of all of the vessels in the body because the point Taiyuan (Lu 9) is located in the *cun* position of the *cun kou;* this is a congregating point for *qi* of the Lung Channel. Since all the Channels of *zang-fu* organs converge in the lung, it is said that all the channels and vessels meet in the lung. Furthermore, the Lung Channel communicates with the Spleen Channel. The spleen and stomach, in turn, are the source of the nutrients that maintain the functioning of all the organs; they are also the source of transformation of *qi* and blood. Accordingly, the pulse at the *cun kou* reflects the condition of the *zang-fu* organs, the channels and vessels, and the *qi* and blood of the entire body.

During pulse-taking, the patient should sit, or lie on his or her back. The room should be quiet, and the patient's *qi* and blood should be calm. The pulse should not be taken soon after physical activity, after drinking, or when the patient has been excited, because these all affect the pulse. In general, the best time for pulse-taking is early in the morning.

The patient's hand should be placed, palm up, on a cushion; the forearm should be at or near the heart level to allow the blood to circulate smoothly. With adults, three fingers are used: first, the middle finger locates the *guan;* then, the index finds the *cun* while the ring finger finds the *chi.* The fingers should arch so that their tips line up and the cushions of the fingers touch the pulse. With children, the thumb alone may be used, since the child's *cun kou* is too short to be divided.

Three readings are taken. For the first, the fingers press gently against the wrist to obtain a superficial sensation; then moderate pressure is applied to obtain a deeper sensation and, finally, heavy pressure, that is, applying with a force that almost stops the pulse beat. The duration of pulse-taking should not be less than one minute for each reading.

The purpose of taking the pulse is to determine any abnormalities in its depth, frequency, rhythm, strength, smoothness, and amplitude. A normal pulse has a frequency of about four to five beats per breath and a regular rhythm. It is even, stable, and forceful. It will vary with physiological and climatic conditions, however. In children, for example, the pulse is usually soft and rapid; in adolescents and adults, it is more forceful; in elderly people, it tends to be weaker.

The female pulse is often softer, weaker, and more rapid than the male pulse. A heavy person tends to have a deep pulse, while a thin person's pulse is "floating." The normal pulse may be slightly taut in spring, full in summer, floating in autumn, and sinking in winter. These are normal variations.

An abnormal pulse is a mirror of pathological changes in the body. Throughout the centuries of practice of traditional Chinese medicine, much medical literature—and lore—has been devoted to the classification and description of abnormal pulse conditions.[22] Today, the standard is the 28-pulse classification; however, only 17 pulse types are common in clinical practice. These types may be viewed as pairs, since they are relative descriptions: a deep pulse, for example, is recognized only by contrast to a floating pulse. The 17 common pulse types may be summarized as follows:

The Floating Pulse and the Deep Pulse

The characteristic of the floating and deep pulse is the depth of location—and hence the amount of pressure necessary to sense the pulse.

The floating pulse is superficial. It responds to the finger when pressed lightly but feels weak when heavy pressure is applied. It indicates an exterior symptom-complex involving primarily the superficial channels of the body. It occurs when the so-called pulse *qi*— that is, the *qi* circulating in the vessels—rises to the surface as the defensive *yang qi* emerges to combat the attacks of pathogenic wind-cold on the body surface. Generally speaking, a floating and forceful pulse indicates an exterior symptom-complex of excess; while a floating and forceless pulse indicates an exterior symptom-complex of deficiency often seen in a mild infectious disease at its early stage. The information of a floating pulse may be related to an increased volume of cardiac output, the dilation of the peripheral vessels and their decreased elastic resistance, and the fullness of the radial artery. These changes can be seen in an infectious disease accompanied by fever.

A deep pulse may be either weak or strong. A deep forceful pulse

22. For example, twenty-four types of pulse were suggested in *The Pulse Classic,* sixteen types in *Jing Yue's Complete Works,* and twenty-seven in *The Pulse Studies of Bin-hu.* A twenty-eighth pulse—the "hasty" pulse—was added in the *Guidebook for Physicians,* by Li Zhongzi (1642).

indicates an interior symptom-complex of excess; its cause is the inner stagnation of *qi* and blood due to the accumulation of pathogenic factors in the interior. A weak deep pulse, on the other hand, indicates an interior symptom-complex of deficiency caused by the sinking of *qi* due to an insufficiency of *yang qi.*

In general, the appearance of a deep pulse signals that: (1) the volume of cardiac output is normal or decreased; and (2) the peripheral vessels are contracted, and their elastic resistance is increased. This condition appears in cases of severe illness or when the body is in a state of stress. Sometimes, however, the pulse may temporarily be deep and tight (see below) in the early stage of an exterior symptom-complex if *yang qi* is "trapped" within the body by exogenous pathogenic factors.

The Slow Pulse and the Rapid Pulse

Abnormalities in the frequency of the beat of the pulse produce either a slow or a rapid pulse. A slow pulse is one with 3 or fewer beats per breath, or fewer than 60 beats per minute. It may be forceful, indicating the accumulation of cold, or without much force, indicating a *yang* deficiency. In the former case, blood circulation is usually impeded by pathogenic cold, phlegm, or blood stasis. However, a slow but forceful pulse may also be the result of a disruption of blood circulation by pathogenic heat. The only way to distinguish which is the cause—heat or cold—is to refer to the other signs and symptoms. Athletes or manual workers often have a slow pulse. This is their normal physiological condition.

The rapid pulse is one with more than 5 beats per breath or more than 90 beats per minutes. It usually occurs together with a smooth pulse and can be mistaken for a smooth pulse. The distinction is frequency. A smooth pulse is fluent but of normal frequency; a rapid pulse has a high frequency. Thus, Li Shizhen warned:

> Never mistake a smooth pulse for a rapid pulse, which can be identified only by its high frequency.
>
> *The Pulse Studies of Bin-hu*

A rapid pulse indicates a symptom-complex of heat. If it is forceful, it suggests the presence of excess heat, usually from exogenous

factors. In this case, the confrontation between the exuberant pathogenic heat in the interior and the abundant *yang qi* of the body
accelerates the blood flow.

If a rapid pulse is without force, the condition is usually one of
heat of the deficiency type. When the body fluid and blood have
been consumed by a prolonged illness such as tuberculosis, a deficiency of vital essence causes a flaring up of deficiency fire and interior heat. This condition is registered by the rapid, forceless pulse.
Patients suffering from heart failure or severe hemorrhaging may also
have a rapid, forceless pulse; however, in these cases, the pulse will
also be thready (see below).

The Empty Pulse and the Full Pulse

The terms "empty" and "full" describe the strength of the throb
of the pulse. The empty pulse can be felt with light, moderate, or
heavy pressure but feels forceless and void to the fingers. It indicates
deficiency of both *qi* and blood: it is forceless because *qi* is insufficient to impel blood flow, and it feels void because the blood is
inadequate to fill the vessels.

Whether slow or rapid, the empty pulse indicates a symptom-
complex of deficiency, and hence a weakening of the body's functions
and its ability to respond to disease. It must be distinguished from
a pulse that is flowing and forceless but feels strong under heavy
pressure; this latter pulse type usually indicates a heat stroke rather
than a deficiency symptom-complex.

A full pulse has full, strong throbs that are perceptible under light,
moderate, and heavy pressure. It points to a symptom-complex of
excess; it is thus an indication that the body is functioning well and
will respond with strength to any disease. The struggle between the
excessive pathogenic factors and the sufficient vital energy produces
an abundance of *qi* and blood, which, in turn, produce the full pulse.

The Slippery Pulse and the Choppy Pulse

The slippery and choppy pulses are said to *run* differently. The
slippery pulse feels smooth and flowing, like beads rolling on a plate.

It usually indicates a mild illness in which *qi* and blood are sufficient and the antipathogenic factor is strong. Typically, the slippery pulse indicates a symptom-complex of excess heat, the accumulation of undigested food, or a symptom-complex of phlegm.[23] It may also appear during pregnancy in women with ample *qi* and blood as well as in healthy people with very strong constitutions.

The choppy pulse feels like an unsmooth flow of blood to the finger. It is fine, short, and slow. The throb of the beat arrives, but not all at once; it falls away, but not immediately. A choppy pulse indicates a stagnation of *qi* or blood, deficiency of blood, or an injury to essence. It is most common in cases of anemia or other debilitated conditions. These conditions occur when the stagnation of *qi* or blood impedes the flow of *qi*. This inhibition of *qi* flow, together with the consumption of essence, means that the vessels are not properly nourished, and anemia results.

The Overflowing Pulse and the Thready Pulse

This pair of pulses is distinguished by the size and momentum of the pulse throb. The overflowing pulse feels large under light pressure. Its beat is likened to dashing waves that rise forcefully and then decline suddenly. It feels similar to the floating pulse—as though it is right at the surface of the wrist—but it is broader and more forceful. It is a sign of excess heat and appears frequently in the second or advanced stages of infectious disease.[24] It may also appear in other illnesses that cause the blood to be hyperactive. The excess internal heat produces dilation of the blood vessels, an exuberance of *qi,* and a surge of blood, all of which produce the sensation that the pulse is overflowing.

As its name implies, the thready pulse is fine; however, it is clearly perceptible under heavy pressure. A thready pulse may occur in a variety of conditions. Healthy people who have been subjected to cold or who are in a state of nervous stress will often have a thready pulse. Most commonly, the thready pulse is a sign of deficiency of

23. The symptom-complex of phlegm describes such conditions as chronic bronchitis, bronchiectasis, or pulmonary emphysema.

24. For a discussion of the stages of disease from the perspective of Chinese medicine, see chapter 6, "Pathogenesis."

qi and blood or of both *yin* and *yang*. A deficiency of blood and *yin*, in particular, will produce a thready pulse.[25] Sometimes, a thready pulse may occur when pathogenic dampness has produced a prolonged injury to the vessels; this is not a deficiency condition but rather one of excess or a complex condition between deficiency and excess.

The Taut Pulse and the Soft Pulse

Differences in tautness and rigidity of the arteries distinguish the taut and soft pulses. To the fingers, the taut pulse gives the sensation of pressing on a violin string. It is rigid and forceful and travels in a long straight wave that can be felt on the three regions of the *cun*, *guan*, and *chi*, as though they were linked by a cord. This type of pulse indicates a disorder of the gallbladder or the retention of phlegm, or a sharp pain.[26]

The soft pulse lacks tension. It is superficial, soft, and fine. It can be felt under light pressure, but it feels forceless and thready. It indicates a symptom-complex of either deficiency or dampness. It occurs in cases of debilitation, when *qi* and blood are insufficient, or in cases of edema.

The Tight Pulse and the Relaxed Pulse

The tight and relaxed pulses differ in tension. The tight pulse is tense and forceful, it feels like a tightly stretched cord. It differs from the taut pulse, which is also cordlike, in that the tight pulse is smaller in size and not so tightly stretched, and not so tense to the finger. The tight pulse is characteristic of symptom-complexes of cold, pain, and the accumulation of food.[27]

25. A thready pulse appears in cases recognized by Western medicine as anemia, reduced blood volume, and various heart diseases such as aortic or mitral stenosis, pericardial effusion, or severe myocarditis.

26. The taut pulse appears to occur in cases of hepatitis, cirrhosis, cholecystitis, hypertension, arteriosclerosis, chronic bronchitis, pulmonary emphysema, duodenal ulcers, menstrual irregularities, cancer of the cervix, and nephritis.

27. The tight pulse may be linked to arthralgia and arteriosclerosis.

The relaxed pulse is loose. Even though the pulse rate is four beats per minute, the relaxed pulse gives the impression of a slow and relaxed movement. It is most common in conditions of pathogenic dampness or weakness of the spleen and stomach. When a patient's pulse becomes relaxed, it is a sign that the body's resistance is being restored.

The Hasty Pulse, the Slow and Uneven Pulse, and the Intermittent Pulse

These three pulses form a set distinguished by missing beats. The hasty pulse is rapid with irregular missing beats. The slow and uneven pulse is slow with irregular missing beats. The intermittent pulse has a moderate frequency, but misses beats at regular intervals. Sometimes, the intermittent pulse is called a "compensatory pulse," since a short beat closely follows each missed beat, as if to replace it.

A hasty pulse indicates excess *yang* and *heat* with a stagnation of blood and *qi*.[28]

A slow and uneven pulse indicates blockage of *qi* due to excess *yin,* cold, phlegm, or blood stasis.[29]

The intermittent pulse signals the functional decline of the *zang* organs. This pulse rhythm is difficult to maintain due to the consumption of *qi* and blood and the deficiency of original *yang* which often underlie it. It usually occurs in cases of severe heart disease. However, it may also occur in cases of strong pains, fever, fright, and injuries such as fractures, contusions, and strains. In these latter cases, it does not indicate a severe condition.

The Multi-Feature Pulse

When disease occurs, several types of pathogenic factors usually attack the body at the same time. Also, the condition of the vital energy as well as the location and nature of pathological changes vary

28. The hasty pulse appears to be common in myocarditis caused by infectious disease and in some types of heart disease.

29. The slow and uneven pulse appears in heart diseases resulting from coronary arteriosclerosis and rheumatic heart disease.

frequently over the course of disease. Accordingly, the types of pulse described above rarely occur in isolation.

Rather, they occur in combination, forming a "multi-feature" pulse. Pairs of opposing pulses—such as the empty pulse and the full pulse— cannot occur together. But all other combinations of pulses are possible. These combinations usually indicate a combination of the conditions indicated by the individual pulses.

For example, a floating pulse indicates exterior disease, while a tight pulse indicates a symptom-complex of cold. Thus, a floating and tight pulse indicates a symptom-complex of cold in the exterior of the body.

A deep pulse indicates interior disease while a slow pulse indicates a symptom-complex of cold. A deep and slow pulse therefore implies a symptom-complex of cold in the interior.

A more complicated example is a deep, thready, and rapid pulse. The deep pulse indicates an interior symptom-complex; the thready pulse, a deficiency; and the rapid pulse, heat. The deep, thready, and rapid pulse is therefore a sign of a symptom-complex of interior heat of the deficiency type.

When the Pulse Contradicts the Symptoms . . .

Generally, the pulse agrees with the symptoms of the patient. Symptoms of excess usually coincide with the presence of a pulse of excess, such as an overflowing, rapid, or full pulse. In these cases, the vital energy is vigorous enough to resist excessive pathogenic factors. Similarly, in prolonged diseases, when the symptoms are weakness and deficiency, the pulse usually feels deep, fine, thready, and/or weak. Although the vital energy is thus insufficient, the pathogenic factor is weakening; there is good hope for recovery.

Sometimes, however, the pulse may contradict the observed symptoms. For example: a deep, thready, or weak pulse may occur in an illness of excess. Or a floating, overflowing, full, or rapid pulse may occur in a prolonged case of weakness and deficiency. In both cases, the prognosis is poor. In the first case, the pathogenic factor is rampant and is about to prevail over the antipathogenic qi. In the second case, the antipathogenic *qi* has declined, while the pathogenic factor remains undiminished. These contradictory pulses and symptoms are signs of the advanced stage of a disease; the condition is a complex one involving symptom-complexes of both excess and deficiency.

A second cause of contradictory pulses and symptoms is the appearance of a false pulse. In this case, the practitioner faces a dilemma: should the diagnosis be based on the pulse or on the symptoms and signs? The stakes are usually high in these cases. For example, when the symptoms and signs of appendicitis have disappeared, a rapid pulse may remain. This pulse usually indicates residual inflammation. Under these circumstances, treatment should be based on the pulse condition, rather than the signs and symptoms, in order to prevent a relapse. On the other hand, an overflowing pulse may indicate an exuberance of *qi* while severe diarrhea or hemorrhaging indicate the opposite. In this case, treatment should be based on signs and symptoms rather than the pulse condition, and therefore, imperative measures are necessary to prevent collapse due to the perishing of *yin* and *yang*.

The answer to this dilemma is that there can be no simple answer. The pulse is an important indicator of the pathological condition of the body and an essential component of the diagnosis. However, it cannot be considered as the only daignostic evidence. Only by analyzing the data gathered from all of the diagnostic methods described in this chapter—and by interpreting them according to the principles for the differentiation of symptom-complexes to be presented in the next chapter—can a comprehensive and correct diagnosis be made.

IN SUMMARY

Traditional Chinese medicine uses four principal methods of examination: looking, listening, asking, and feeling.

Looking is the visual inspection of the body. Such an inspection can reveal much about the body, according to Chinese medicine, since the condition of the interior is reflected on the exterior. Looking includes inspection of the physique, the facial expression, the color of the complexion, the secretions and excretions of the body, and the features of the head and face. Perhaps most important, however, is the inspection of the tongue: its color, shape, surface condition, and type of coating all provide specific information about the type of illness and the efforts of the body to reestablish a normal, healthy state.

Listening is a method of gathering information about the body from the sounds of the voice, breathing, and digestive system.

Asking is the process of determining the patient's chief complaint as well as past history and life style. The guide to this process is the so-called "Ten Questions," which inquire about chills and fever; perspiration; pain in the head, trunk, and limbs; sensations in the chest and abdomen; defecation and urination; appetite; thirst; hearing; previous history of disease; and the onset of the present illness.

Feeling includes palpation of the trunk and limbs as well as pulse-taking. Of these two, pulse-taking is the more highly developed method. Chinese medicine recognizes seventeen types of pulses that can occur alone or in combination. These pulse types play a central role in diagnosis.

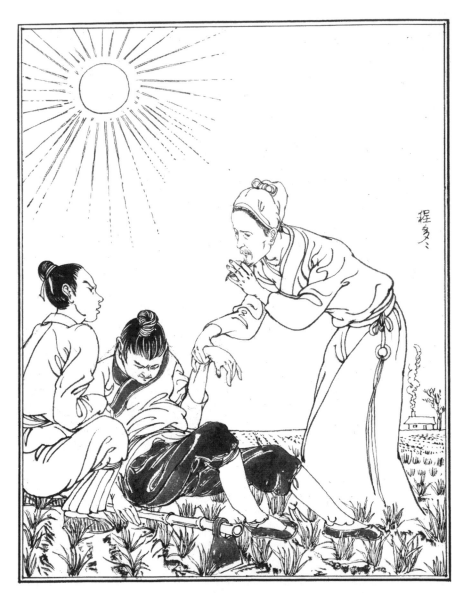

A rural worker has fainted from being exposed to the sun too long.

CHAPTER EIGHT

Diagnosis:
The Differentiation of
Symptom-Complexes

THE DIFFERENTIATION OF symptom-complexes is the key to diagnosis and treatment in traditioanl Chinese medicine.

Symptom-complexes are a way of classifying pathological symptoms and signs to determine the basic disharmony in the body. Each symptom-complex is a set of signs and symptoms that can be observed through the various diagnostic methods described in chapter 7. It identifies the origin, location, and nature of the disease.

The main goal in differentiating among symptom-complexes is to identify changes in the functioning of the body and to understand the characteristics of the disease. This goal corresponds to the view that illness is always the result of two factors: (1) the antipathogenic factor, which produces changes in the functioning of the body to maintain a healthy balance of *yin* and *yang;* and (2) the pathogenic factor, which has a characteristic path of development.

Understanding these two factors is more important in Chinese medicine than seeking the cause of a disease or the underlying organic changes. This emphasis is also practical: the functional changes that both patients and practitioners observe are usually more prominent and obvious than changes in the morphology and structure of the body. At the same time, the functional changes present a portrait of the pathological changes, which occur according to regular laws.

Each symptom-complex is thus a detailed picture of the condition of the body.

A diagnosis based on symptom-complexes may change over the course of the illness. Symptom-complexes do not describe diseases. They describe the functioning of the body *at a definite time and stage of a disease.* The condition of the body is constantly changing as the pathogenic and antipathogenic factors confront each other—as the body struggles to maintain a dynamic equilibrium between its internal condition and the external environment. Accordingly, the symptoms and signs of an illness will change as it proceeds, and so must the diagnosis of symptom-complexes.

While the symptom-complex does not describe an entire disease, it does describe the influence of the disease on the entire body. Each symptom-complex embodies an understanding of the relationship among functions in the body and of the pathological changes that can occur in those relationships. If a symptom-complex is properly recognized and treated, the treatment should restore harmony to the body's functions. The integrity of the body will not be violated by the treatment.

In the course of the history of traditional Chinese medicine, a variety of methods for classifying signs and symptoms into symptom-complexes has evolved. These different methods are sometimes based on different theories or take different systems within the body as their starting point. Taken together, however, they define a general approach to diagnosis. In this approach, symptom complexes are differentiated accordint to:

- the "Eight Guiding Principles"
- the state of *qi* and blood
- the theory of the *zang-fu* organs
- the theory of the Six Channels
- the general theory of the channels
- the theory of the *wei, qi, ying,* and *xue* systems
- the theory of the Triple Burner
- the etiology of disease

Most important among these methods is differentiation according to the "Eight Guiding Principles." The Eight Principles are *yin* and *yang,* interior and exterior, cold and heat, deficiency and excess. Signs and symptoms of a disease are classified according to these eight categories. The remaining methods are used to refine this basic diagnosis.

Not all methods apply to all conditions. Thus, the process of differentiating symptom-complexes proceeds in stages. First, the condition will be classified in one of two categories: exterior symptom complexes of infectious disease due to exogenous pathogenic factors; or interior symptom complexes of internal disorders.

Symptom complexes of the first category may be further differentiated according to the theories of the Six Channels, the Triple Burner, and the *wei, qi, ying,* and *xue* systems. Those of the second category must be analyzed according to the state of *qi* and blood, the *zang-fu* theory, and the general theory of the channels. Finally, whether the condition belongs to the first or second category, it may be further interpreted according to the theory of etiology.

For example, the practitioner begins by attempting to grasp the main symptoms. These will invariably be the chief complaints of the patient or the most obvious signs and symptoms of the patient. (They should not be considered the main symptoms throughout the entire course of the disease, however.) The practitioner then determines whether the condition is an exterior condition resulting from exogenous pathogenic factors or an interior condition due to internal disorders. If the disease is due to exogenous pathogenic factors, the practitioner must ask whether it is due to cold or heat. All of this is done according to the Eight Guiding Principles.

Now, if the disease is due to exogenous cold, the practitioner continues to analyze the condition according to the theory of the Six Stages of Cold-Induced Diseases. If the condition is due to exogenous heat, further analyses are based on the theories of *wei, qi, ying,* and *xue* or of the Triple Burner.

On the other hand, if the practitioner determines that the condition is an interior symptom-complex, the next step (which is still part of the method of differentiation according to the Guiding Principles) is to determine whether it is a deficiency or excess condition. Deficiency symptom-complexes are further differentiated according to the state of *qi* and blood. In addition, the *zang-fu* organs and the channels where the disease is located must be identified. For example, the condition may be one of deficiency of heart *qi* or blood, or of a disorder in the Shaoyin or Taiyin Channels.

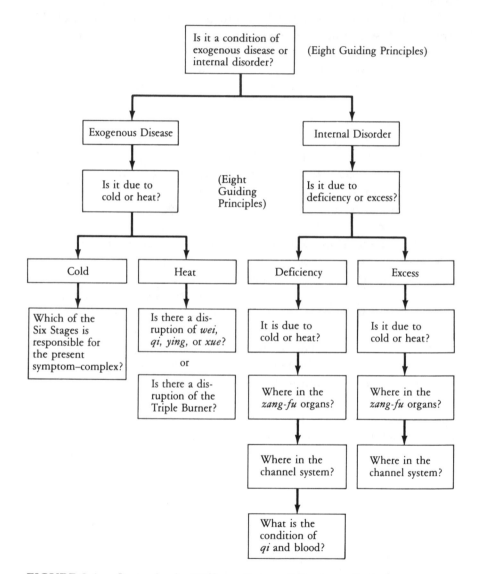

FIGURE 8.1. **Stages in the Differentiation of Symptom-Complexes**

Excess symptom complexes are differentiated primarily according to the location of the disease in the *zang-fu* organs and in the channels.

Figure 8.1 outlines these stages of analysis. The specific details of each stage as well as the symptom-complexes associated with each method are the subject of the remaining pages of this chapter.

THE EIGHT GUIDING PRINCIPLES

The foundation for the Eight Guiding Principles originated in the *Classic of Internal Medicine* (475–221 B.C.) and was reorganized during the Ming Dynasty (1368–1644) by the distinguished physician Zhang Jingyue. Zhang introduced the idea of differentiating the "six changes" by integrating the theories of etiology, of the *zang-fu* organs, of *qi* and blood, and of the Six Channels. In the Qing Dynasty (1644–1911), Cheng Zhongling expanded Zhang's "changes" into a comprehensive system for differentiating symptom-complexes. The "six changes" were categorized according to their *yin* or *yang* nature; thus, the system of Eight Guiding Principles became the theoretical basis for treatment of disease in traditional Chinese medicine.

As already indicated, the eight principles, or parameters, are:

- *yin* and *yang,* which describe the general type of disease
- interior and exterior, which describe the location of the disease
- cold and heat, which describe the specific nature of the disease
- deficiency and excess, which describe the state of the struggle between antipathogenic *qi* and the pathogenic factor

Of these, *yin* and *yang* are the most comprehensive. *Yang* symptom-complexes include exterior, heat, and excess symptom-complexes; *yin* symptom-complexes include interior, cold, and deficiency symptom-complexes. Because they are the most comprehensive, however, the *yin* and *yang* are too general to be differentiated directly. They are determined only after the other six Principles have been interpreted.

The evaluation of the eight principles thus follows a step-wise procedure as follows:

INTERIOR OR EXTERIOR?

⇔

COLD OR HEAT?

⇔

DEFICIENCY OR EXCESS?

⇔

YIN or YANG?

This procedure allows a complex analysis of the condition of the body. But it leads to an evaluation that can be simply stated: namely, that the disease is either essentially a *yin* condition or a *yang* condition.

Differentiating Exterior and Interior Symptom Complexes

Exterior and interior are the principles that describe the location of the disease. They also suggest the direction of the development of the disease.

Interior refers to the *zang-fu* organs. Interior symptom-complexes may result from transmission of exogenous pathogenic factors to the interior if they are not eliminated in time. Or they may indicate internal disorders of the organs due to abnormal emotions, irregular food intake, excessive strain or stress, excess or lack of physical excercise. These symptom-complexes are usually more severe and appear in the more advanced stages of a disease.

Exterior and interior symptom-complexes are the *systemic response* of the body to pathogenic factors. Therefore, they are not differentiated by the anatomical parts of the body that are affected, but rather by a set of general symptoms that have come to be associated with exterior and interior conditions: these include chills and fever, tongue coating, the condition of the pulse, and the degree of functional disturbance in the *zang-fu* organs.

Exterior and interior symptom-complexes may be differentiated by the following characteristics:

EXTERIOR SYMPTOM-COMPLEXES. These are usually benign. They are marked by sudden onset and are short-lived. The major distinguishing symptoms are an aversion to cold (or wind) and a thin, white coating on the tongue.

Exterior-symptom complexes typically occur in the early stages of an infectious disease. They signal a defensive response to the pathogenic factors or toxins in the body. While the entire body responds, there is no severe malfunctioning of the organs, systems, or energy metabolism.

INTERIOR SYMPTOM-COMPLEXES. These are more serious and arise in one of three ways: (1) exogenous pathogenic factors that have not been treated in time are transmitted to the interior and the situation is transformed into an interior symptom-complex; (2) the organs are invaded directly by exogenous pathogenic factors, such as interior cold due to over consumption of raw or cold foods; and (3) functional disturbances occur in the organs as a result of deficient functioning due to emotional disturbances.

The characteristic signs of interior symptom-complexes are fever with no aversion to cold or an affinity for warmth, restlessness, delirium, palpitations, pain and distension in the abdomen, a sensation of weakness in the lower back and knees, scanty and concentrated urine, constipation or loose stools, a yellow tongue coating or the absence of a tongue coating, and a deep pulse. Such symptom-complexes typically appear in the advanced stages of disease. (They may signal major disturbances of the nervous system of Western medicine as well as the metabolism of energy.) Functional disturbances of the organs are common in chronic cases.

(In differentiating interior and exterior symptom-complexes, it is important to note these distinctions: an interior symptom-complex may be accompanied by an aversion to cold, but this aversion will be relieved by warm clothing; in an external symptom-complex, the cold feeling will not be alleviated by warm clothing. Similarly, the fever in interior symptom-complexes occurs at regular intervals and is accompanied by an intolerance of heat; the fever of an exterior symptom-complex is irregular and is often accompanied by an aversion to cold. Furthermore, if the disease progresses from the exterior to the interior, both the interior and the exterior may be affected. Or pathogenic cold may re-attack the body. Both of the above situations will produce a confusion of symptoms.)

SYMPTOM-COMPLEXES OF BOTH THE EXTERIOR AND THE INTERIOR. These may coexist. There are two cases of this condition: the first is a simultaneous disturbance of both the exterior and the interior; the second is the transmission of exogenous pathogenic factors to the interior without the elimination of the exterior condition.

SYMPTOM-COMPLEXES OF A DISTURBANCE BETWEEN THE EXTERIOR AND THE INTERIOR. These appear when a disease that was initially an exterior infectious disease advances toward the interior. The exterior symptom-complex may not disappear before the interior

TABLE 8.1.   Differentiation of Cold, Heat, Deficiency, and Excess in Exterior Symptom-Complexes

The basic symptoms of exterior symptom-complexes are aversion to cold (or wind) and a thin white tongue coating. Other symptoms are fever, headache and general aching, nasal obstruction, a floating pulse, and sometimes coughing and asthma.

Symptom-Complex	Chief Symptoms for Differentiation	Approach to Treatment
Cold in the exterior	Severe aversion to cold and a slight fever Severe headache and general aching Thin, moist, and white tongue coating Floating and forceful pulse	Dispel pathogenic factors from the exterior of the body with sudorifics pungent in flavor and warm in nature
Heat in the exterior	High fever with moderate aversion to cold Dry throat and thirst Thin and dry tongue coating Reddened tongue Floating and rapid pulse	Dispel pathogenic factors from the exterior of the body with drugs pungent in flavor and cool in nature
Exterior deficiency	Aversion to wind Profuse perspiration Floating and slow pulse	Adjust the *wei* and *ying* systems
Exterior excess	Absence of sweating General aching Stiff neck Floating and forceful pulse	Dispel pathogenic factors from the exterior of the body with sudorifics pungent in flavor and warm in nature

symptom-complex appears. In this case, the condition is said to be one of both the exterior and the interior. Such symptom-complexes are typical of malaria, infections of the biliary and urinary tracts, and pancreatitis. The chief symptoms of this condition are: alternating spells of chills and fever; a bitter taste and dryness in the mouth;

TABLE 8.2. Differentiation of Cold, Heat, Deficiency, and Excess in Interior Symptom-Complexes

The basic symptoms of interior symptom-complexes are fever; irritability; palpitations, wheezing; distending pain in the stomach and abdomen; soreness and weakness in the lumbar region; disorders in the elimination of wastes; a yellow tongue coating or the absence of a tongue coating; delirium or unconsciousness; deep pulse.

Symptom-Complex	Chief Symptoms for Differentiation	Approach to Treatment
Cold in the interior	Pallor/ Aversion to cold/ Cold limbs and a preference for heat/ Preference for hot beverages/ Expectoration of thin sputum/ Diarrhea accompanied by abdominal pain/ Pain and spasm in the testes/ Clear profuse urine/ Pale tongue with white or white and smooth coating/ Deep and slow pulse	Use warming methods
Heat in the interior	Flushed face/ Fever and chills/ Thirst, restlessness, and perspiration/ Preference for cold beverages/ Deep yellow scanty urine/ Constipation, foul-smelling diarrhea or bloody stools containing pus/ Deep-red tongue with yellow coating/ Overflowing and rapid pulse	Use febrifugal methods
Interior deficiency	General lassitude/ Feeble breathing/ Apathy/ Vertigo and palpitations/ Loss of appetite/ Loose stools/ Flabby and pale tongue with white coating or absence of coating/ Deep and weak pulse	Use tonifying methods
Interior excess	Restlessness/ Coarse breathing/ Constipation/ Distending pain in the abdomen/ Aggravated by pressure/ Delirium or mania/ Thick, yellow tongue coating/ Deep and full pulse	Use purgative methods

TABLE 8.3.   Differentiation of Symptom-Complexes of Both the Exterior
and Interior

Symptom-Complex	Chief Symptoms for Differentiation
Cold in both the exterior and interior	Aversion to cold Headache and general aching Pain in the abdomen Diarrhea Cold limbs White and smooth tongue coating Deep and tight pulse
Heat in both the exterior and interior	Persistent fever Headache Flushed face Dry throat and thirst Restlessness Red tongue with thin, yellow coating Overflowing and rapid pulse
Deficiency in both the exterior and interior	Spontaneous perspiration Intolerance of wind Dizziness Palpitations Weak voice Diarrhea Pale tongue with smooth coating Weak or irregular, intermittent pulse
Excess in both the exterior and interior	Aversion to cold Fever without perspiration Headache and general aching Distending pain in the abdomen aggravated by pressure Dysfunction in urination and bowel movement Thick, white and slimy tongue coating Full pulse or taut, slippery pulse
Cold in the exterior and heat in the interior	Aversion to cold Fever and absence of perspiration Restlessness Thirst Red tongue with thin, yellow coating Floating, tight and rapid pulse
Heat in the exterior and cold in the interior	Fever without perspiration Headache and coughing Loose stools and clear urine

Symptom Complex	Chief Symptoms for Differentiation
	Flabby tongue with light, yellow coating
	Deep and taut pulse
Deficiency in the exterior and excess in the interior	Spontaneous perspiration and intolerance of wind
	Distending pain in the abdomen
	Fullness in the chest
	Nausea
	Constipation
	Thick, white and slimy tongue coating
	Floating and slippery pulse
Excess in the exterior and deficiency in the interior	Aversion to cold
	Absence of perspiration
	Headache and general aching
	Shortness of breath
	Incontinence of urine
	Absence of thirst
	Flabby tongue with thin, white coating
	Floating and weak pulse

nausea and vomiting; distending pain in the chest and costal region; pain and a feeling of choking in the stomach; loss of appetite, and a taut and rapid pulse.

With the exception of a symptom-complex of both the exterior and interior, all of these symptom-complexes must be further differentiated according to cold and heat and deficiency and excess. Tables 8.1–8.3 summarize the main differentiating symptoms and the method of treatment for each of these. In addition, the diagnosis of interior symptom-complexes depends not only on these other parameters, but also on the condition of the Six Channels; the condition of the *wei, qi, ying,* and *xue* systems; and the strength of the pathogenic factors.

Differentiating Symptom-Complexes of Cold and Heat

Cold and heat are the principles that identify the specific nature of a disease. Cold symptom-complexes are provoked by pathogenic cold or by hypofunctioning and a preponderance of *yin* due to insufficiency of *yang.* Heat symptom-complexes result from a hyperfunctioning and preponderance of *yang* due to pathogenic heat or such pathological changes as fire arising from stagnant *qi* and heat resulting from accumulated *yang* in the five *zang* organs.

In addition to simple cold and heat symptom-complexes, there may appear symptom-complexes of coexisting and interlocking cold and heat, true cold with pseudoheat, and true heat with pseudocold. These may be differentiated as follows:

COLD SYMPTOM-COMPLEXES. These are characterized by a lowered body temperature, intolerance of cold and preference for heat, absence of thirst (or preference for sips of hot beverages,) loose stools, clear profuse urine, a pale tongue with a white coating, and a slow, deep, fine, or weak pulse. Cold limbs, listlessness, and pallor are also characteristic.

In the early stages of an infectious disease, symptoms such as aversion to cold, fever, absence of perspiration, and a floating and tight pulse also indicate cold in the exterior. (See table 8.1.)

HEAT SYMPTOM-COMPLEXES. These may be recognized by fever, an aversion to heat; flushed face; irritability; a preference for cold beverages; concentrated urine; constipation or yellow, sticky, and foul-smelling stools; a burning sensation in the anus; a reddened tongue with a dry yellow coating; and a rapid, overflowing, and forceful pulse.

A heat symptom-complex does not necessarily involve a fever. In the absence of fever, key symptoms are thirst, a dry throat, constipation, urine with a reddish tinge, a red tongue with a yellow coating, and a rapid pulse.

CO-EXISTING AND INTERLOCKING COLD AND HEAT. This indicates the simultaneous appearance of both cold and heat symptom-complexes. Such conditions may occur in functional disturbances of the alimentary tract. When cold and heat symptom-complexes co-exist, one-half typically appears in the upper body while the other appears in the lower body. Table 8.4 summarizes the differences in cold and heat in the upper and lower body.

A SYMPTOM-COMPLEX OF TRUE COLD WITH FALSE HEAT. This indicates that an internal abundance of *yin* is hindering *yang* from

TABLE 8.4.   Differentiation of Cold and Heat in the Upper and
Lower Body

Location of Cold and Heat	*Chief Symptoms for Differentiation*
Cold in the upper body	Sour regurgitation and belching/ Dyspepsia/ Fullness in the epigastrium and abdomen
Cold in the lower body	Abdominal pain, relieved by pressure and warmth/ Loose stools/ Incontinence of urine/ Cold legs and feet
Heat in the upper body	Distending sensation in the head/ Headache/ Red eyes/ Toothache/ Sore throat/ Dry mouth and preference for cold beverages
Heat in the lower body	Constipation/ Concentrated urine with dark, yellow tinge/ Pain in the urethra

the outside (see chapter 6.) This symptom-complex occurs during the most advanced stage of a disease and indicates that the patient is critically ill.

The chief symptoms are: a feverish sensation of the body; a flushed face, thirst, involuntary restless movement of the limbs, and an overflowing, but forceless pulse. Further observation, however, reveals cold symptoms such as the need for warm clothing and heavy bedding when the fever is present and listlessness. The patient also feels thirsty but has no desire to drink or prefers hot beverages. Other cold symptoms that appear are clear urine, loose stools, a white coating on the tongue, and overflowing but forceless pulse.

A SYMPTOM-COMPLEX OF TRUE HEAT WITH FALSE COLD. This is also a critical condition. It is caused by a preponderance of internal heat that obstructs the release of *yin*. The symptoms are: pallor, cold limbs, and a deep, thready pulse, all of which resemble a cold symptom-complex. Further observation, however, reveals that the patient has no desire for warm clothing or heavy bedding, even though his or her limbs are cold. Typically, there is also a hot burning sensation in the chest and abdomen. While the pulse is deep and fine, it is also forceful. Other typical heat symptoms are also present: thirst, a dry throat, a preference for cold beverages, concentrated urine, and constipation. (As these descriptions suggest, the key factors in determining true or false cold and heat are: forcefulness of the pulse, color and moistness of the tongue, presence or absence of thirst, preference for cold or hot beverages, color of urine, preference for warm clothing and bedding, and the sensation of either cold or heat in the chest and abdomen.)

Symptom-complexes of cold and heat must be further differen-

TABLE 8.5.   Differentiation of Deficiency and Excess in Cold and Heat Symptom-Complexes

Symptom-Complex	Chief Symptoms for Differentiation	Approach to Treatment
Excess cold	Aversion to cold/ Cold limbs/ Distending pain and coldness in the abdomen/ Constipation/ Wheezing/ Fullness in the chest/ Livid face and lockjaw in severe cases/ White, slimy tongue coating/ Deep, hidden pulse or taut, tight pulse	Dispel internal cold with drugs warm in nature; relieve constipation
Deficiency cold	Intolerance of cold/ Cold limbs and affinity for warmth/ Diarrhea with watery stools containing undigested food/ Clear and profuse urine/ Listlessness/ Pallor/ Pale and flabby tongue/ Slow, thready, and weak pulse	Warm *yang* and reinforce vital energy
Excess heat	Continuous high fever/ Restlessness and thirst/ Delirium/ Fullness and distending pain in the abdomen aggravated by pressure/ Reddened tongue with yellow coating/ Overflowing, rapid, slippery, and full pulse	Eliminate pathogenic heat
Deficiency heat	Afternoon fever/ Night sweats/ Gaunt form and lassitude/ Feverish sensation in the palms, soles, and heart area/ Dry throat and mouth/ Reddened tongue with little coating/ Fine and rapid pulse	Replenish *yin* and eliminate pathogenic heat

tiated according to deficiency and excess. Deficiency is most common in cases of cold symptom-complexes; chronic cases and cases of gastrointestinal dysfunction or heart failure are typical examples. They indicate decline in physiological functions, a decrease in energy metabolism, or a weak resistance to fever.

Excess is most common in heat symptom-complexes. Such conditions are typical in infectious diseases or diseases that produce an increase in energy metabolism (such as hyperthyroidism.) They indicate a hyperfunctioning of the body and a strong response to pathogenic factors.

Although the typical pattern for cold and heat symptom-complexes is deficiency with cold and excess with heat, the reverse may also appear. Excess cold symptom-complexes are usually due to pathogenic cold and the retention of undigested food, leading to dysfunction in the gastrointestinal system. They may also result from obstruction of lung *qi* by cold phlegm. Deficiency heat symptom-complexes are due primarily to excessive consumption of essence and blood, to the failure of *yin* to check *yang,* and to hyperfunctioning of the deficiency type (see chapter 6.) The key symptoms for differentiating deficiency and excess in cold and heat symptom-complexes appear in table 8.5.

Differentiating Symptom-Complexes of Deficiency and Excess

Deficiency and excess describe the struggle between antipathogenic *qi* and the pathogenic factors. They characterize: (a) the response of the human body to the pathogenic factor; (b) the strength and weakness of the antipathogenic and pathogenic factors in the course of their confrontation; and (c) hypo- or hyperfunctioning of the organs and other body systems.

Deficiency is a condition in which the body's resistance is lowered and its functions are weak. In the extreme, deficiency may result in collapse.

Excess denotes a condition in which the pathogenic factor is hyperactive while the antipathogenic *qi* is still strong enough to produce a severe struggle between the two. It also refers to pathological conditions characterized by the accumulation of fluids and the formation of lumps.

Like symptom-complexes of cold and heat, those of deficiency and
excess can occur simultaneously. Also, conditions of false-deficiency
and false-excess can appear. The major distinguishing features of each
of these types of symptom complexes are:

DEFICIENCY SYMPTOM-COMPLEXES. These typically occur in chronic
diseases. They may also occur during the stage of recovery from acute
infectious diseases. The symptoms of deficiency symptom-complexes
vary greatly; however, they may be classified into four basic types:
deficiency of *yin,* deficiency of *yang,* deficiency of *qi,* and deficiency
of blood.

A deficiency symptom-complex should be suspected if the patient
shows: pallor or a sallow complexion, listlessness, gaunt appearance,
general lassitude, heart palpitations, weak voice, insomnia, amnesia,
spontaneous sweating or night sweats, chills and cold limbs, a feverish sensation in the palms, soles, and the area of the heart, incontinence of feces and urine, pain that can be relieved by pressure, a pale
tongue with a thin coating or no coating, and a fine and weak pulse.

EXCESS SYMPTOM-COMPLEXES. These are provoked by two factors:
(1) hyperactivity of exogenous pathogenic factors in the body or (2)
a functional disorder of the organs or metabolic system that results
in the accumulation and stagnation of pathological products such as
phlegm, dampness, and blood stasis from abnormal internal bleeding.

Because of the variety of possible pathogens and of possible locations of the disease, the diseases of excess vary greatly. However, the
chief indicators of an excess symptom-complex are: an appearance of
physical strength, nervous excitement, a sonorous voice, high fever,
a feeling of fullness and distending pain in the abdomen that is aggravated by pressure, a suffocating feeling in the chest, and irritability. In severe cases, the symptoms may also include: delerium, coarse
breathing, excessive phlegm and saliva, constipation or the urgent
sensation of needing to defecate or urinate, difficulty in urination, a
thick coating on the tongue, and an overflowing and forceful pulse.

The key factors in distinguishing deficiency and excess symptom-
complexes are thus: the strength of the physical appearance, signs of
vitality, the sound of the patient's breathing, the effect of pressure
on areas that are painful, and the condition of the tongue and pulse.

SYMPTOM-COMPLEXES OF SIMULTANEOUS DEFICIENCY AND EX-
CESS. These can occur when the antipathogenic *qi* is weak and thus
fails to contend with the pathogenic factor in the course of the disease. For example, a patient may suffer from coughing, with frequent
expectoration of sticky sputum and a thick yellow tongue coating;
all of these symptoms indicate an excess symptom-complex due to
obstruction of the lung by heat and sputum. At the same time,
however, the patient may demonstrate symptoms of deficient lung
qi, such as shortness of breath and wheezing when active. This is a
symptom-complex of both excess and deficiency.

Another example is a case in which internal bleeding results in
abdominal lumps, indicating an excess symptom-complex. Yet the
same patient may also show signs of deficiency of blood: a gaunt
form, dry scaly skin, and darkness around the eyes. Such cases indicate a persistent hypofunctioning of antipathogenic *qi* together with
an excess symptom of lumps.

A SYMPTOM-COMPLEX OF TRUE EXCESS AND FALSE DEFICIENCY.
This appears when conditions of true excess cause obstruction of the
channels and stagnation of *qi* and blood. Typical of these conditions
are accumulated heat in the stomach and intestines, the accumulation
of phlegm and undigested food, or the formation of abdominal masses.
By obstructing channels, they bring about listlessness, chills, cold
limbs, and a deep, slow pulse or a deep, hidden pulse, all of which
suggest deficiency symptom-complexes. If examined closely, however, patients with these conditions will have a sonorous voice and
coarse breathing. While the pulse is deep and slow, it is also forceful. These suggest that the phlegm, undigested food, and heat are
the main cause of the disease and that the deficiency symptoms are
false-symptoms.

SYMPTOM-COMPLEXES OF TRUE DEFICIENCY AND FALSE EXCESS.
These occur when conditions of deficiency due to inadequate *qi* and
blood in *zang-fu* organs and impaired transport and transformation of
body substances create excess symptom-complexes. These are characterized by a feeling of fullness and distending pain in the abdomen
and a taut pulse. Closer examination will reveal that the feeling of
fullness is not always present and that the abdominal pain may be
relieved by pressure. While the pulse is taut, it feels forceless under

pressure. The latter signs indicate that the true nature of the disease is insufficient *qi* and blood and impaired transport and transformation.

Differentiating Symptom-Complexes of Yin *and* Yang

As already mentioned, *yin* and *yang* are general parameters that encompass the other six parameters. Thus, symptom-complexes of exterior, heat, and excess conditions are classified as *yang* symptom-complexes, while those of interior, cold, and deficiency conditions are *yin* symptom-complexes.

In addition, the parameters of *yin* and *yang* also describe some of the pathological changes of the *zang-fu* organs. When Chinese medicine speaks of symptom complexes of *yin* deficiency or *yang* deficiency and of perishing *yin* or perishing *yang,* it is specifically referring to the condition of the *zang-fu* organs.

In general, *yin* symptom-complexes are characterized by a weakening of *yang* in the body, a stagnation of pathogenic cold due to hypofunctioning, a decrease in energy metabolism, and insufficient heat. Blood diseases and disorders of the *zang* organs are also *yin* symptom-complexes.

Yang symptom-complexes are characterized by a preponderance of internal heat and *yang qi* due to hyperfunctioning, an increase in energy metabolism, and excessive heat. Typically, *qi* disorders and disturbances of the *fu* organs are considered *yang* diseases.

The primary factor in these symptom-complexes is an imbalance between *yin* and *yang*. The nature of their pathological changes are simply characterized as *yin* or *yang*. However, some symptom-complexes may result from a basic imbalance of *yin* or *yang,* when one fails to check the other due to the consumption of either vital essence or vital energy. These produce the symptom-complexes of *yin* or *yang* deficiency, which may be described as follows:

SYMPTOM-COMPLEXES OF *YIN* DEFICIENCY. These are characterized by two types of symptoms: (1) a gaunt appearance, a dry mouth, the absence of a tongue coating, and a fine pulse all suggest insufficient vital essence; (2) a feverish sensation in the palms, soles, and region of the heart; fever in the afternoon, night sweats, a deep red tongue; and a fine rapid pulse all indicate the growth of internal pathogenic heat of the deficiency type.

Yang Deficiency Symptom-Complexes. These are characterized by: (1) listlessness, lassitude, apathy, weak voice, lying with the body curled up, somnolence, and a feeble pulse, all of which indicate a deficiency of vital energy and hypofunctioning; and (2) an intolerance of cold, cold limbs, a diminished sense of taste, absence of thirst, clear urine or reduced amounts of urine with a full sensation, pallor, and a pale tongue, which all suggest an increase of internal cold of the deficiency type and an exuberance of damp-cold in the interior.

A Symptom-Complex of Perishing Yin. This indicates the collapse of vital essence due to massive consumption of body fluids. It is usually brought on by extreme heat, conditions of severe deficiency, massive hemorrhaging, or excessive vomiting.

A Symptom-Complex of Perishing Yang. This indicates a severe impairment and collapse of vital energy. Extreme cold, conditions of severe *yang* deficiency, or profuse sweating can each cause a perishing of *yang*.

TABLE 8.6.   Differentiation of Symptom-Complexes of Perishing *Yin* and *Yang*

Symptom-Complex	Chief Symptoms for Differentiation	Approach to Treatment
Perishing of *yin*	Sticky sweating/ Shortness of breath and rapid breathing/ Hot skin and warm hands and feet/ Irritability/ Preference for cold beverages/ Flushed face/ Reddened and dry tongue/ Fine and rapid pulse	Nourish *yin* and reinforce vital energy
Perishing of *yang*	Profuse cold sweating/ Feeble breathing/ Cool skin and limbs/ Listlessness/ Lying with the body curled up/ Absence of thirst or preference for hot beverages/ Pallor/ Pale and moist tongue/ Thready and fading pulse	Rescue *yang* from collapse

The last two symptom-complexes—those of perishing *yin* and *yang*—are critical conditions. The body's *yin* and *yang* are mutually supporting. The perishing of *yin* thus results in a dispersion of *yang* since *yang qi* has nothing to support it; the perishing of *yang* leads to an exhaustion of vital essence due to failure in the functions of transport and transformation. Emergency aid is necessary in these cases.

Table 8.6 lists the distinguishing symptoms and treatments of the *yin* and *yang* symptom-complexes.

THE STATE OF *QI* AND BLOOD

In cases of endogenous disorders, a more complex theory of the state of *qi* and blood is used in making a diagnosis. This theory distinguishes several types of disorders of *qi,* of blood, and and of both *qi* and blood.

For example, there are four types of disorders of *qi:*

—Deficiency of *qi* is a symptom-complex in which there is a hypo-functioning of the organs or of one individual organ; it is common in chronic conditions, during stages of recovery from acute diseases, and during general recovery by old, weak patients.

—Sinking of *qi* is a symptom-complex in which a deficiency of *qi* occurs, marked by a failure in the support of tissues due to the weakness of *qi*. It is typical of cases of prolapse of internal organs, such as the stomach, kidney, or uterus.

—Stagnation of *qi* is a symptom-complex characterized by the blockage of *qi* in a certain part of the body or in an individual organ. This blockage impedes the flow of *qi,* producing conditions recognized in Western medicine, including such disorders as endocrine disturbances, premenstrual tension, hepatitis, and ulcers.

—Adverse flow of *qi* is a symptom-complex that indicates a disturbance in either the upward or downward functions of the body. It includes dysfunctions in moving food downward. More typically, however, it refers to upward or adverse functioning of the lungs, stomach, and liver as well as to an exuberance of liver *yang*. This symptom-complex is typical of infections of the upper respiratory tract, pneumonia, gastritis, and hypertension.

TABLE 8.7.　Differentiation of Symptom-Complexes According to the State of *Qi*

Symptom-Complexes	Chief Symptoms for Differentiation	Treatment
Deficiency of *qi*	Lack of strength to breathe and speak/ Apathy/ General lassitude/ Dizziness/ Spontaneous sweating that is worse when active/ Pale tongue/ Empty pulse	Reinforce *qi* with tonics
Sinking of *qi*	Lack of strength to breathe/ Lassitude/ Distension and a sensation of bearing-down in the abdomen/ Prolapse of rectum or uterus/ Pale tongue/ Empty pulse	Reinforce *qi* to restore ability to uplift
Stagnation of *qi*	Suffocating feeling and pain	Remove obstruction of *qi*
Adverse flow of *qi*	Coughing/ Asthma/ Belching/ Hiccups/ Nausea/ Vomiting/ Headache/ Dizziness/ Fainting or hematemesis in severe conditions	Bring down the upward *qi* to correct its adverse flow

Table 8.7 summarizes the key characteristics in differentiating these symptom-complexes.

While there are many symptom-complexes that involve disorders of the blood, they may be grouped into three general classes.:

—Deficiency of blood denotes those symptom-complexes in which the blood fails to nourish the vessels due to the decreased quality of blood. Anemia is the most common example.

—Stagnancy of blood indicates a disturbance in blood circulation due primarily to a disorder in an individual organ. It is common in cardiovascular diseases, cerebrovascular accidents, enlargement of the liver and spleen, disorders of the uterus, menstrual irregularities, tubal pregnancy, and postpartum disorders.

—Noxious heat in the blood system occurs when pathogenic heat invades the blood system. It is typical of eruptive infectious dis-

TABLE 8.8.   Differentiation of Symptom-Complexes According to the
State of Blood

Symptom-Complexes	Chief Symptoms for Differentiation	Treatment
Deficiency of blood	Pallor or sallow complexion/ Pale lips/ Dizziness/ Palpitations and insomnia/ Numbness of the hands and feet/ Pale tongue/ Empty pulse	Tonify the blood
Stagnancy of blood	Pains, Masses/ Hemorrhaging/ Hemorrhagic spots due to bleeding in the tissues/ Dark complexion and darkened skin around the eyes/ Dry scaly skin/ Dark-red tongue/ Fine and choppy pulse	Remove blood stasis by promoting blood circulation
Noxious heat in the blood system	Restlessness/ Mania/ Coma/ Deep-red tongue/ Rapid pulse/ Various kinds of hemorrhaging with massive amounts of red or dark-red blood/ Purpura	Dispel pathogenic heat from the blood system with drugs cool in nature

eases such as measles, scarlet fever, epidemic meningitis, and other hemorrhagic diseases.

Table 8.8 outlines the chief features of these symptom-complexes.

A variety of symptom-complexes involve disorders of both *qi* and blood. These include:

- Stagnation of both *qi* and blood
- Deficiency of both *qi* and blood
- Deficiency of *qi* and loss of blood
- Prostration of *qi* after great loss of blood
- Deficiency of *qi* and stagnation of blood
- Stagnation of blood and deficiency of blood

These symptom-complexes are summarized in table 8.9.

TABLE 8.9.   Differentiation of Symptom-Complexes According to
Disorders of Both the *Qi* and Blood

Symptom-Complexes	*Chief Symptoms for Differentiation*	*Treatment*
Stagnancy of *qi* and blood	Fullness and distending pain in the chest and stomach region/ Irritability/ Presence of a painful mass aggravated by pressure/ Amenorrhea/ Dysmenorrhea with discharge of dark-red blood and blood clots/ Distending pain in the breast	Invigorate blood circulation by regulating the flow of *qi*
Deficiency of *qi* and stasis of blood	General lassitude/ Feeble breathing/ Spontaneous sweating/ Pain aggravated by pressure/ Dark tongue with red surface spots	Reinforce *qi* to promote blood circulation
Deficiency of both *qi* and blood	Lack of strength to breathe and speak/ Lassitude/ Spontaneous sweating/ Pallor or sallow complexion/ Palpitations and insomnia/ Pale and flabby tongue/ Thready and weak pulse	Reinforce *qi* and tonify blood
Deficiency of *qi* and loss of blood	Hemorrhaging (subcutaneous bleeding and uterine bleeding in women)/ Shortness of breath/ General lassitude/ Pallor/ Pale tongue/ Fine and weak pulse	Reinforce *qi* to keep blood flowing within the vessels
Prostration of *qi* after great loss of blood	Massive hemorrhaging associated with pallor/ Cold limbs/ Profuse sweating/ Fainting/ Feeble and thready or hollow pulse	Reinforce *qi* to prevent collapse
Stagnancy of blood and deficiency of blood	Dizziness/ Palpitations and insomnia/ Pale tongue with red spots on it/ Fine and choppy pulse/ Painful masses that appear in fixed spots and are aggravated by pressure	Invigorate blood circulation and nourish blood

THE *ZANG-FU* ORGANS

The theory of the *zang-fu* organs provides a strong foundation for classifying symptom-complexes that result from internal disorders. According to this theory, each of the organs performs a distinct physiological function and is subject to different pathological changes. When the functioning of an organ is disrupted, it will therefore produce a distinctive symptom-complex.

At the same time, however, there is a set of relationships between each *zang* and *fu* organ and between the *zang-fu* organs and other tissues of the body. All of these are also described by the theory of the *zang-fu* organs. The basic task of the practitioner is to identify the pathological changes associated with the individual *zang* or *fu* organs while keeping in mind the interrelationships and mutual influence among all of the organs. The following descriptions of symptom-complexes illustrate this process.

The Heart and Small Intestine

The main physiological functions of the heart are governing the blood and controlling mental activities. Pathological changes of the heart thus appear as disturbances of blood circulation and mental activities. These may be conditions of either excess or deficiency. They include:

—Deficiency due to inadequate heart *yang* or heart *qi* is common in cases of functional heart disease and some organic heart disease, in failures of the peripheral circulation, in anemia, and in some illnesses of weakness.
—Deficiency due to inadequate heart *yin* or heart blood appears in cases of anemia and some organic heart diseases.
—Excess due to a flaring up of heart fire is typical of glossitis.
—Excess due to stagnation of heart blood and obstruction of the vessels describes the condition found in cases of coronary arteriosclerosis, including angina pectoris and myocardial infarction.
—Excess due to phlegm and fire in the heart characterizes mental disturbances such as hysteria, schizophrenia, and epilepsy.
—Excess due to obstruction of the Heart Channel by phlegm is typical of comas due to cerebrovascular accidents.

The distinguishing characteristics of these symptom-complexes are outlined in table 8.10.

The *fu* organ related to the heart is the small intestine. Its principal function is to digest and differentiate the usable from the nonusable. Disorders of the small intestine thus appear primarily as disturbances in digestion and failures of the body to differentiate usable substances from nonusable, including some pathological changes in the urinary system. The typical symptom-complexes are:

—Deficiency due to hypofunction and cold is usually seen in cases of intestinal spasm and enteritis, among others.
—Excess due to damp-heat in the small intestine is typical of infections of the urinary system, including cystitis, urethritis, and prostatitis.
—Excess due to the stagnation of *qi* in the small intestine describes the condition of an inguinal hernia.

Table 8.11 differentiates these symptom complexes.

The Lung and Large Intestine

The lung controls *qi* and respiration. It also regulates the dispersion of *qi* to keep the passageways of water unobstructed. A diseased lung may be recognized by dysfunctions of respiration. Lung problems should also be suspected in cases of attack by exogenous wind, cold, heat, and dryness. There are seven symptom-complexes of the lung:

—Deficiency of lung *qi* may occur in chronic bronchitis, pulmonary emphysema, and pulmonary tuberculosis, for example.
—Deficiency of lung *yin* may also occur during recovery from pneumonia, and other lung infections.
—Excess due to invasion of the lung by wind-cold is typical of upper respiratory tract infections, acute and chronic bronchitis, bronchial asthma, and pulmonary emphysema.
—Excess due to invasion of the lung by wind-heat may also occur in upper respiratory tract infections, in acute bronchitis, pneumonia, and pulmonary abscess, and acute tonsilitis and pharyngitis.
—Excess due to invasion of the lung by pathogenic dryness is typi-

TABLE 8.10. Differentiation of Symptom-Complexes of the Heart

Symptom-Complex		General Symptoms	Chief Symptom-Complexes for Differentiation	Treatment
Deficiency	Deficiency of heart *qi*	Palpitations/ Dyspnea/ Spontaneous sweating that is worse when active	Pallor/ General lassitude/ Pale tongue with thin coating/ Fine, weak, or irregular intermittent pulse	Tonify heart *qi*
	Deficiency of heart *yang*		Pallor/ Chills/ Cold limbs/ Cardiac retardation/ Fullness in the chest/ Pale or dark-red tongue/ Fine, weak or irregular intermittent pulse	Tonify heart *yang*
	Deficiency of heart blood	Sleep disturbed by dreams/ Palpitations/ Amnesia/ Insomnia	Sallow complexion/ Dizziness/ Pale lips/ Pale tongue/ Fine pulse	Tonify heart blood
	Deficiency of heart *yin*		Restlessness/ Feverish sensation in the palms and soles/ Afternoon fever/ Night sweats/ Dry mouth/ Reddened tongue with little saliva/ Thready, rapid pulse	Nourish heart *yin*

Excess			
	Flaring up of heart fire	Ulceration of the mouth and tongue/ Swelling and pain of the tongue/ Restlessness/ Insomnia/ Dry mouth/ Dark yellow urine/ Red tongue tip/ Rapid pulse	Remove intense heat from the heart by purging the fire
	Stagnation of heart blood and obstruction of the vessels	Palpitations/ Paroxysmal fullness or stabbing pain in the heart and chest arising in the shoulder and back/ Cold limbs/ Sweating/ Cyanosis of lips and nails in severe cases/ Dark-red tongue or purple spots on the tongue/ Choppy or irregular intermittent pulse	Activate blood circulation by removing obstruction of vital energy and reinforce function
	Mental disturbance due to phlegm and fire	Restlessness/ Insomnia/ Dream-disturbed sleep in mild cases/ Mental disorders/ Weeping and laughing without reason/ Mania in severe cases/ Reddened tongue with yellow slimy coating/ Taut, slippery and forceful pulse	Expel stubborn phlegm and purge fire
	Obstruction of the heart channel by phlegm	Mental restlessness/ Delirium/ Mania/ Coma/ Sound of phlegm in throat/ White, slimy phlegm in throat/ White, slimy tongue coating/ Slippery pulse	Expel stubborn phlegm and resuscitate

TABLE 8.11.   Differentiation of Symptom-Complexes of the Small Intestine

Symptom-Complexes	Common Symptoms for Differentiation	Treatment
Hypofunction of the small intestine due to cold	Pain in the lower abdomen relieved by pressure and heat/ Frequent nausea/ Loss of appetite/ Loose stools/ Flabby pale tongue/ Deep and fine pulse	Invigorate *yang* to dispel cold
Damp-heat in the small intestine	Restlessness/ Difficulty in urination accompanied by scanty urine and with reddish tinge/ Pain in the urethra/ Frequency and urgency of urination or blood in urine/ Distending pain in the umbilicus and abdomen/ Red tongue with yellow coating/ Slippery and rapid pulse	Eliminate damp heat with febrifugal and diuretic drugs
Painful hernia of the small intestine	Lateral prolapse of inguinal hernia with pain that is eased when lying supine/ Borborygmus/ White tongue with smooth coating/ Taut and slippery pulse	Promote the normal flow of *qi* to remove stagnation and pain

cal of the common cold in autumn; it also may appear in cases of bronchitis.

—Excess due to retention of phlegm-heat in the lung appears most frequently in cases of chronic bronchitis, secondary infections of bronchiectasis, pneumonia, and pulmonary abscess.

—A symptom-complex of excess due to blockage of the lung by phlegm-dampness is typical of bronchial asthma, bronchiectasis, pulmonary emphysema, and chronic asthmatic bronchitis.

These symptom-complexes and their chief symptoms are summarized in table 8.12.

The large intestine, which is related to the lung, conveys solid wastes from the body. Any dysfunction in the elimination of solid wastes therefore suggests pathological changes in the large intestine. These may be of the following types:

—Deficiency due to insufficient fluid in the large intestine is typical of habitual constipation or constipation after childbirth.

—Incontinence due to deficiency of *qi* in the large intestine ap-

TABLE 8.12.   Differentiation of Symptom-Complexes of the Lung

Symptom-Complex			Symptom-Complexes for Differentiation	Treatment
Deficiency	Deficiency of lung *qi*	Cough	Cough/ Asthma/ Lassitude/ Shortness of breath/ Feeble voice/ Intolerance of cold/ Spontaneous sweating/ Pallor/ Expectoration of copious thin sputum/ Pale tongue with white coating/ Empty and weak pulse	Reinforce lung *qi*
	Deficiency of lung *yin*		Dry cough or cough with sticky sputum scanty in amount/ Blood tinged sputum/ Dry mouth and throat/ Afternoon fever/ Night sweats/ Malar flush/ Feverish sensation in palms, soles and the heart area/ Reddened tongue with thin coating/ Fine and rapid pulse	Nourish *yin* and moisten the lung
Excess	Invasion of the lung by wind-cold	Headache and cough	Aversion to cold/ Fever/ Headache and general aching/ Watery nasal discharge/ Expectoration of mucoid sputum/ White coating/ Floating and tight pulse	Ventilate and smooth the troubled lung and dispel cold
	Invasion of lung by wind-heat		Cough/ Headache/ Fever/ Aversion to wind/ Thirst/ Sore throat/ Expectoration of thick yellow sputum/ Thin yellow coating/ Floating and rapid pulse	Ventilate and smooth the troubled lung with drugs pungent in flavor and cool in nature

TABLE 8.12.   *(Continued)*

Symptom-Complex			Symptom-Complexes for Differentiation	Treatment
Excess (cont.)	Invasion of lung by pathogenic dryness	Headache and cough (cont.)	Dry cough with scanty sputum/ Difficulty in expectoration due to thick sputum/ Asthmatic cough/ Expectoration of white frothy sputum/ Dry throat and nose/ Chest pain in severe cough/ Fever/ Aversion to wind-cold/ Dry tongue with thin coating little saliva/ Fine rapid pulse	Clear up the lung to relieve dryness
	Retention of phlegm-heat in the lung		Asthmatic cough/ Coarse breathing/ Expectoration of thick, yellow sputum or foul purulent sputum speckled with blood/ Pain in chest/ Sore throat/ Thirst/ Constipation/ Scanty urination with reddish tinge/ Reddened tongue with yellow coating/ Rapid pulse	Dispel and disperse the lung's heat
	Blockage of the lung by phlegm-dampness		Cough with expectoration of copious sputum or thin, white frothy sputum/ Rasping in the throat/ Difficulty in lying supine/ Pale tongue with white, slimy coating/ Slippery pulse	Eliminate dampness by drying, regulate the flow of *qi* and dissolve phlegm

pears in cases of prolapse of the rectum, chronic dysentery, and enteritis.

—Excess due to damp-heat in the large intestine often occurs in acute enteritis, acute bacillary dysentery, amoebic dysentery, or acute attacks of chronic dysentery.

—Excess due to the accumulation of dryness in the large intestine appears when the intestine is obstructed.

—Excess due to the accumulation of heat in the large intestine describes the condition of appendicitis.

Table 8.13 differentiates these symptom-complexes.

The Spleen and Stomach

The spleen transports nutrients and maintains blood within the vessels. Pathological changes in the spleen thus appear as dysfunctions in digestion and the assimilation of nutrients, as well as hemorrhaging due to the failure of the spleen to control blood. Stagnation of water and dampness also indicates problems with the spleen. As with the other organs, symptom-complexes of the spleen may be conditions of deficiency or excess:

—Deficiency of spleen *qi* often appears in chronic enteritis, dysfunctions of the stomach and intestines, intestinal tuberculosis, malnutrition, and inability to assimilate nutrients.

—Deficiency due to a sinking of spleen *qi,* occurs in cases of prolapse of the rectum, uterus, and other organs.

—Deficiency due to the failure of the spleen to control blood describes many cases of hemorrhaging, including functional uterine bleeding, bleeding hemorrhoids, and thrombopenic purpura.

—Deficiency of spleen *yang* occurs in cases of ulcers, chronic gastritis, chronic enteritis, chronic nephritis, and general dysfunctions of the stomach and intestines. It also describes edema due to malnutrition and conditions of excessive vaginal discharge.

—Excess due to invasion by cold-dampness occurs in acute enteritis and diarrhea with large amounts of undigested food.

—A symptom-complex of excess due to damp-heat in the spleen and stomach may be seen in the jaundice of acute hepatitis and also in diarrhea where large amounts of food have not been digested.

TABLE 8.13. Differentiation of Symptom-Complexes of the Large Intestine

Symptom-Complex		Chief Symptoms for Differentiation	Treatment
Deficiency	Insufficient fluid in the large intestine	Constipation/ Dry stools/ Dry mouth with little saliva/ Reddened tongue with dry or yellow coating/ Fine and choppy pulse	Moisten the large intestine to relieve constipation
	Incontinence due to deficiency of *qi* in the large intestine	Persistent dysentery/ Defecation accompanied by gas or incontinence of feces/ Prolapse of the rectum/ Cold limbs/ Dull pain in the abdomen that is relieved by heat and pressure/ Pale tongue with white coating/ Slow and weak or deep and feeble pulse	Administer styptic drugs to treat incontinence or treat incontinence of feces and strengthen the rectum
Excess	Damp-heat in the large intestine	Pain in the abdomen/ Tenesmus/ Dysentery with pus and blood/ Excretion of thin, yellow water in large amounts/ Burning sensation of the anus/ Scanty urination with reddish tinge/ Reddened tongue with yellow slimy coating/ Slippery and rapid pulse	Eliminate heat and dampness with febrifugal and diuretic drugs
	Accumulation of dryness in the large intestine	Constipation/ Fullness and distending pain in the abdomen, aggravated by pressure/ Nausea/ Vomiting/ Yellow white slimy tongue coating or yellow and dry coating/ Taut and slippery pulse	Remove heat and promote bowel movement by use of purgatives cold in nature
	Blockage of the large intestine by accumulated heat	Distension in the epigastrium and fullness in the abdomen/ Pain in the right lower abdomen aggravated by pressure/ Constipation or mild diarrhea/ Fever/ Concentrated urine/ Yellow slimy tongue coating/ Taut pulse	Activate blood circulation to remove blood stasis and remove heat and constipation by use of purgatives

Table 8.14 summarizes these symptom-complexes.

The function of the stomach is to take in and digest food. When the stomach is functioning normally, stomach *qi* is always descending. If signs of ascending stomach *qi* or dyspepsia appear, the stomach is disturbed. Such disturbances may take the following forms:

—Deficiency of stomach *yin* may occur in chronic gastritis, ulcers, gastroneurosis, diabetes, and in the advanced stages of an infectious disease.

—Excess due to hyperactivity of stomach fire is typical in some infectious diseases that are accompanied by high fever, in chronic or acute gastritis, in stomatitis, in periodontitis.

—Excess due to retention of food in the stomach describes the condition of dyspepsia.

Table 8.15 summarizes the distinctive features of these symptom-complexes of the stomach.

The Liver and Gallbladder

The liver governs the smooth flow of *qi;* it stores blood and controls the condition of the tendons. Failures in any of these functions indicate liver trouble and lead to the following symptom-complexes:

—Deficiency of liver blood may occur in anemia, peripheral neuritis, and inadequate menstrual flow or failure to menstruate.

—Excess due to the depression of liver *qi* appears typically in chronic hepatitis, chronic cholecystitis, and neurosis.

—Excess due to flaring up of liver fire is characteristic of hypertension, neuralgic headache, hemorrhaging in the upper alimentary tract, and acute conjunctivitis.

—Excess due to exuberance of liver *yang* is typical in hypertension, various menopause syndromes, and neurosis.

—Excess due to endogenous wind stirring may take one of three forms: (1) liver *yang* turning to wind; (2) stirring of wind in the liver due to extreme heat; and (3) endogenous growth of wind in the liver due to blood deficiency. These symptom-complexes appear in cases of hypertension, cerebral arteriosclerosis, cerebrovascular accidents, and convulsions due to high fever.

—Excess due to dampness and heat in the liver and gallbladder may

TABLE 8.14. Differentiation of Symptom-Complexes of the Spleen

Symptom-Complex		General Symptoms	Chief Symptoms for Differentiation	Treatment
Defi-ciency	Deficiency of spleen *qi*		Feeble breathing/ Apathy/ Gaunt form/ General lassitude/ Fullness in the abdomen after meals/ Pale tongue with white coating/ Slow and weak pulse	Reinforce *qi* and tonify the spleen
	Sinking of spleen *qi*	Poor appetite/ Fullness and distension in the abdomen/ Loose stools/ Pallor or sal-low complex-ion	Distension and a bearing-down sensa-tion in the stomach region, epigas-trium and abdomen/ Dyspnea/ Tenes-mus/ Prolapse of rectum and uterus or other organs/ Gastroptosis/ Pale tongue/ Weak pulse	Reinforce *qi* to restore ability to uplift
	Failure of the spleen to control blood		Bloody stools/ Blood in urine/ Exces-sive menstrual flow/ Uterine bleeding/ Purpura/ Pale tongue/ Weak pulse	Reinforce *qi* and control blood

	Deficiency of spleen *yang*	Chills/ Cold limbs/ Dull pain in the stomach region and abdomen relieved by pressure and heat/ Pale tongue with white coating/ Deep and slow pulse	Warm the spleen and stomach to dispel cold
	Invasion of the spleen by cold	Nausea/ Tastelessness in the mouth/ Absence of thirst/ Abdominal pain/ Diarrhea/ Heaviness of the head/ Lassitude/ Edema/ White slimy tongue coating/ Soft and relaxed pulse	Warm the spleen and stomach, dispel dampness and tonify the spleen
Excess	Damp-heat in the spleen and stomach	Nausea/ Poor appetite/ General sluggishness/ Loose stools/ Difficult urination with reddish tinge/ Yellow complexion of the sclera, skin/ Stickiness and sweet taste in the mouth/ Yellow slimy tongue coating/ Soft and rapid pulse	Remove heat and eliminate dampness

TABLE 8.15. Differentiation of Symptom-Complexes of the Stomach

Symptom-Complex		Chief Symptoms for Differentiation	Treatment
Defi-ciency	Insufficiency of stomach *yin*	Dry mouth and lips/ Hunger without increased eating/ Stom-achache/ Belching/ Nausea/ Dry stools/ Reddened tongue with lit-tle saliva/ Fine and rapid pulse	Nourish stomach *yin*
Excess	Hyperactivity of stomach fire	Burning sensation with pain in the stomach region/ Vomiting/ Thirst/ Preference for cold bever-ages/ Hunger/ Foul breath/ Gin-gival swelling, ulceration, and bleeding of gums/ Constipation/ Scanty urination with reddish tinge/ Reddened tongue with yellow coating/ Slippery and rapid pulse	Remove stomach fire by use of purgatives
	Retention of food in the stomach	Distending pain in the stomach region and abdomen/ Vomiting/ Foul belching and sour regurgita-tion/ Poor appetite/ Constipation/ Diarrhea/ Thick and slimy coat-ing of tongue/ Slippery pulse	Promote diges-tion and re-tained food

occur in acute icteric hepatitis, acute cholecystitis, cholelithiasis, abscesses of the liver, cervicitis, and vaginitis.

—Excess due to stagnated cold in the liver channel is typical of chronic orchitis, epididymitis, and hernia.

These symptom-complexes are differentiated in table 8.16.

Diseases often occur in the liver and gallbladder simultaneously. Thus dysfunctions of the liver should suggest possible trouble in the gallbladder and vice versa. One symptom-complex is, however, spe-cifically related to disease in the gallbladder:

—Depression of gallbladder *qi* occurs when there is excess phlegm in the gallbladder. The chief symptoms are: dizziness, nausea, a bitter taste in the mouth, insomnia due to irritability, sensitivity to light, distension in the chest, sighing, a thick and smooth tongue coating, and a taut and slippery pulse. This disorder is characteristic of hysteria and neurosis. The aim of treatment is to

TABLE 8.16. Differentiation of Symptom-Complexes of the Liver and Gallbladder

Symptom-Complex		Chief Symptom-Complexes for Differentiation		Treatment
Deficiency	Deficiency of liver blood	Dizziness/ Dryness of eyes/ Blurred vision/ Night blindness/ Numbness of limbs/ Spasm of tendons/ In women, scanty menstrual flow or amenorrhea/ Pale tongue/ Fine pulse		Nourish liver blood
Excess	Depression of liver *qi*	Pain in the costal region, irritability	Emotional depression/ Suffocating feeling in the chest/ Pain in the hypochondriac region/ Loss of appetite/ Belching/ Distending pain in the stomach region and abdomen/ A sensation of foreign body in the throat/ Menstrual irregularity/ Distending sensation in the breast/ Goiter or masses in the abdomen/ Thin white tongue coating/ Taut pulse	Restore the normal functioning of a depressed liver
	Flare-up of liver fire		Distending pain in the head/ Dizziness/ Irritability/ Flushed face/ Red eyes/ Bitter taste in the mouth/ Dry throat/ Ringing in the ears/ Burning pain in the costal-region/ Hematemesis/ Epistaxis/ Constipation/ Urination with reddish tinges/ Reddened tongue with yellow coating/ Taut and rapid pulse	Quench fire in the liver

TABLE 8.16.   *(Continued)*

Symptom-Complex		Chief Symptom-Complexes for Differentiation		Treatment
Excess (cont.)	Exuberance of liver *yang*	Dizziness/ Ringing in the ears/ Distending pain in the head/ Flushed face/ Red eyes/ Irritability/ Insomnia/ Dream-disturbed sleep/ Amnesia/ Palpitation/ Soreness and weakness in the lumbar region and knee joints/ Reddened tongue/ Taut and rapid pulse		Nourish *yin* and subdue hyperactivity of the liver
Endogenous wind stirring in the liver	Liver *yang* turning to wind	Tremor, spasm, and vertigo	Headache/ Dizziness/ Numbness and trembling of the limbs/ Unconsciousness/ Tongue rigidity that impairs the ability to speak/ Facial paralysis/ Hemiplegia/ Reddened tongue/ Taut and rapid pulse	Subdue hyperactivity of the liver and endogenous wind
	Stirring of wind in the liver by extreme heat		High fever/ Coma/ Convulsion/ Neck rigidity/ Staring of the eyes upward/ Opisthotonos in severe cases/ Reddened tongue with yellow coating/ Taut and rapid pulse	Clear up pathogenic heat, cool the liver and subdue the endogenous wind
	Endogenous growth of wind in the liver due to blood deficiency		Dizziness/ Blurred vision/ Sallow complexion/ Numbness of the limbs/ Trembling/ Spasm of the tendons and muscles/ Tics/ Itchy skin/ Pale tongue/ Taut and fine pulse	Nourish blood and subdue the endogenous wind

Symptom-Complex	Chief Symptom-Complexes for Differentiation	Treatment
Dampness and heat in the liver & gall- bladder	Distending pain in the costal region/ Bitter taste in the mouth/ Poor appetite/ Nau- sea/ Fullness in the abdomen/ Irregular defecation/ Scanty urination with reddish tinges/ Yellow eyes, sclera, and skin/ Scrotum eczema/ Swelling and burning pain of the testes/ Yellow morbid leukor- rhea/ Itching of the vulva/ Yellow slimy tongue coating/ Taut and rapid pulse	Remove dampness and heat from the liver and gall- bladder
Cold stagnated in the liver channel	Distending pain and a bear- ing-down sensation of the lower abdomen and the testes/ Contraction of the scrotum aggravated by cold and eased with heat/ Chills and cold limbs/ White smooth tongue coating/ Deep and taut pulse	Warm the liver and dispel cold

restore normal gallbladder functions to assist the downward move- ment of stomach *qi*.

The Kidney and Urinary Bladder

The kidney stores vital essence, regulates water circulation and the inspiratory phase of respiration and determines the condition of the bones. When it is diseased, the kidney may lose its ability to main- tain vital essence and inspiration; the body will experience problems in growth, development, and reproduction. All symptom-complexes of the kidney are deficiency conditions:

—Deficiency of kidney *yang* is characteristic of adreno-cortical hypo- functioning, hypothyroidism, chronic nephritis, nephrotic syn- drome, and sexual dysfunction.

—Deficiency of kidney *yin* typically occurs in pulmonary tuberculosis, diabetes, diabetes insipidus, nerve deafness, and infertility.
—Deficiency due to the failure of the kidney to promote inspiration may appear in senile bronchitis, bronchiectasis, pulmonary emphysema, and corpulmonale.
—Deficiency due to unconsolidated kidney *qi* is typical of childhood bedwetting, diabetes insipidus, chronic nephritis, and hypofunctioning in sexual activity.
—Deficiency of kidney essence characterizes cases of poor development, infertility, and sexual dysfunction.

Table 8.17 outlines the origins, symptoms, and treatments of these symptom-complexes.

Since the principal functions of the urinary bladder are to store and discharge urine, any abnormality of urination indicates a problem of this organ. The primary symptom-complex of this organ is one of excess:

—Excess due to damp-heat in the urinary bladder can be recognized by frequent urination and an urgent need to urinate; burning pain in the urethra; interrupted urination; turbid urine; blood in the urine; urine stones, accompanied by fever; aching in the lumbar region; distension and fullness in the lower abdomen; a yellow, slimy tongue coating; and a slippery rapid pulse. This symptom-complex is characteristic of urinary system infections, stones, and acute prostatatis. The aim of treatment is to eliminate heat and dampness and restore normal urination.

Symptom-Complexes of More Than One Organ

There are a variety of symptom-complexes that describe conditions involving two of the *zang-fu* organs simultaneously. They include:

• Discord between the heart and kidney, most often seen in neurosis
• Deficiency of both the heart and spleen usually seen in anemia, neurosis, and organic cardiopathy
• *Yin* deficiency of both the lung and kidney usually seen in active pulmonary tuberculosis

TABLE 8.17. Differentiation of Symptom-Complexes of the Kidney and Urinary Bladder

Symptom-Complex		Chief Symptoms for Differentiation	Treatment
Deficiency	Deficiency of kidney *yang*	Pallor/ Chills and cold limbs/ Spontaneous sweating/ Impotence/ Infertility/ Leukorrhea/ Dizziness/ Ringing in the ears/ Pale tongue with white coating/ Deep and fine pulse	Warm kidney *yang* to invigorate the vital function
	Deficiency of kidney *yin*	Dizziness/ Ringing in the ears/ Insomnia/ Amnesia/ Gaunt form/ Dry mouth and throat/ Feverish sensation in the palms, soles, and heart area/ Afternoon fever/ Night sweats/ Malar flush/ Nocturnal emission/ Scanty menstrual flow/ Amenorrhea/ Uterine bleeding/ Reddened tongue with thin dry coating/ Fine and rapid pulse	Nourish kidney *yin*
	Failure of the kidney in promoting inspiration	*Qi* exhaled more than that inhaled/ Dyspnea/ Asthmatic breathing more pronounced when active/ Feeble voice/ Sweating during coughing/ Puffiness of the face/ Pale tongue/ Empty pulse	Warm the kidney to invigorate inspiration
		Soreness and a sensation of weakness over the waist and knees eased by pressure	
Unconsolidated kidney *qi*		Frequent and profuse urine/ Dribbling after urination/ Incontinence of urine/ Frequent urination at night/ Spermatorrhea/ Watery leukorrhea/ Habitual miscarriage/ Pale tongue with white coating/ Deep and weak pulse	consolidate kidney *qi*
Insufficiency of kidney essence		Slow development of infants/ Premature senility/ Loss of hair/ Loosened teeth/ Sluggishness/ Slow movement/ Infertility in men due to low sperm count/ Infertility in women due to amenorrhea/ Reddened tongue/ Fine and rapid pulse	Reinforce kidney essence

TABLE 8.18.   Symptom-Complexes of More Than One Organ

Symptom-Complexes	Symptoms	Treatment
Discord between the heart and kidney	Palpitations/ Amnesia/ Restlessness/ Insomnia/ Dizziness/ Tinnitus/ Dry Throat/ Soreness and a weak sensation in the waist and knees/ Dream-disturbed sleep/ Spermatorrhea/ Afternoon fever/ Night sweats/ Reddened tongue/ Fine and rapid pulse	Nourish *Yin* and eliminate fire to restore the coordination between the heart and kidney
Deficiency of both the heart and spleen	Palpitations/ Amnesia/ Insomnia/ Dream-disturbed sleep/ Poor appetite/ Abdominal distension/ Loose stools/ General lassitude/ Sallow complexion/ Subcutaneous hemorrhaging/ Light-colored menstrual flow/ Uterine bleeding/ Scanty menstruation/ Amenorrhea/ Pale tongue with white coating/ Soft and fine pulse	Tonify the heart and spleen
Yin deficiency of both the lung and kidney	Cough with scanty sputum or blood-streaked sputum/ Dry mouth and throat/ Hoarseness/ Soreness and a weak sensation in the waist and knees/ Restlessness/ Insomnia/ Fever due to deficiency of *yin,* afternoon fever/ Night sweats/ Malar flush/ Spermatorrhea/ Irregular menstruation/ Reddened tongue with thin coating/ Thready and rapid pulse	Moisten and tonify the lung and kidney
Yang deficiency of the spleen and kidney	Aversion to cold, cold limbs/ Soreness and a weak sensation in the waist and knees/ Cold and pain in the lower abdomen/ Pallor or sallow complexion/ Poor appetite/ General lassitude/ Loose stools or dawn diarrhea/ Puffiness of the face and edema of the lower extremities/ Difficulty in urination/ Ascites/ Pale tongue with white coating/ Deep and thready pulse	Tonify the spleen and kidney with drugs warm in nature
Qi deficiency in the spleen and kidney	Shortness of breath/ Lassitude/ Cough with mucoid sputum/ Asthma/ Poor appetite/ Abdominal	Tonify the lung and kidney

Symptom-Complexes	Symptoms	Treatment
	distension/ Loose stools/ Lassitude/ Puffiness of the face and edema of lower extremities/ Pale tongue with white coating/ Thready and weak pulse	
Disharmony between the liver and the spleen	Distending pain and fullness in the chest and rib cage/ Emotional depression/ Irritability/ Poor appetite/ Abdominal distension/ Loose stools/ Borborygmus and flatus/ White or slimy tongue coating/ Taut pulse	Restore the normal functioning of the depressed liver and tonify the spleen
Disharmony between the liver and the stomach	Distending pain and fullness in the chest and ribcage/ Hiccup and belching/ Sour regurgitation/ Emotional depression/ Restlessness/ Irritability/ Thin and yellow tongue coating/ Taut pulse	Restore the normal function of the depressed liver and regulate the stomach function
Deficiency of the kidney and hyperactivity of liver *qi*	Soreness and a weak sensation in the waist and knees/ Spermatorrhea/ Dizziness/ Headache/ Blurred vision/ Tinnitus/ Amnesia/ Irritability/ Flushed face/ Feverish sensation in the palms, soles and heart area/ Reddened tongue/ Taut and fine pulse	Nourish the liver and subdue hyperactivity of liver *qi*
Yang deficiency of the heart and kidney	Chills and cold limbs/ Palpitations, especially continuous violent palpitations/ Oliguria/ Edema/ Cyanosis of lips and nails/ Dark purplish tongue with white smooth coating/ Deep and feeble pulse	Tonify the heart and kidney with drugs hot in nature
Qi deficiency in the heart and lung	Palpitations/ Shortness of breath/ Cough and asthma/ Spontaneous sweating and lassitude, which are both more pronounced when active/ Pallor or sallow complexion/ Cyanosis of lips and nails in severe conditions/ Pale tongue or purple spots on the tongue/ Fine and weak pulse	Tonify the heart and lung

- *Yang* deficiency of the spleen and kidney seen in chronic enteritis, intestinal tuberculosis, chronic nephritis, nephrotic syndrome
- *Qi* deficiency in the spleen and kidney, which typically occurs in chronic bronchitis, complicated by pulmonary emphysema and in pulmonary tuberculosis
- Disharmony between the liver and the spleen, which occurs in gastrointestinal neurosis, chronic enteritis, chronic hepatitis
- Disharmony between the liver and the stomach, which is characteristic of chronic gastritis, gastric dysfunction, chronic cholecystitis, and chronic hepatitis
- Deficiency of the kidney and hyperactivity of liver *qi,* which appears in cases of hypertension, and chronic hepatitis
- *Yang* deficiency of the heart and kidney, which appears most commonly in heart failure and cardiac edema
- *Qi* deficiency of the heart and lung, which is typically seen in pulmonary emphysema and corpulmonale

Table 8.18 lists the chief symptoms of these conditions and the appropriate approach to their treatment.

THE SIX CHANNELS

The theory of the Six Channels, sometimes called the Six Stages, provides a method for further differentiating symptom-complexes that arise due to exogenous pathogenic factors, primarily exogenous cold.[1]

As explained in chapter 4, the channel system includes six pairs of channels that are distinguished by their position, front to back, on the body and by their connection to either a *zang* or a *fu* organ. These six pairs are known as:

—Taiyang
—Yangming
—Shaoyang
—Taiyin
—Shaoyin
—Jueyin

1. This method is based on the *Discussion of Cold-Induced Diseases* and was developed by Zhang Zhongjing during the period of the Eastern Han Dynasty (A.D. 25–220). It is sometimes called the Six Stages or the Six Pairs of Channels.

TABLE 8.19. Differentiation of Symptom-Complexes in Accordance with the Theory of the Six Channels

Channel	Symptom-Complexes		Chief Symptoms for Differentiation	Approach to Treatment
Taiyang	Symptom-complex of the channel	Exterior deficiency (affection by wind)	Aversion to wind Fever Headache Sweating Thin, white tongue coating Floating and slow pulse	Dispel pathogenic factors from the superficial muscles and remove pathogenic wind from the exterior of the body
		Exterior excess (affection by cold)	Aversion to cold Fever Rigidity and pain in the neck General aching Pain in the lumbar region and joints Absence of perspiration Cough and asthmatic breathing Thin, white tongue coating Floating and tight pulse	Dispel pathogenic factors from the exterior of the body by inducing perspiration
	Symptom-complex of the *fu* organs	Retention of fluid in the body	Fever Aversion to wind Sweating Difficulty in urination Thirst Thin, white tongue coating Floating pulse	Promote normal flow of *yang qi* and remove dampness through diuresis

TABLE 8.19. (Continued)

Channel	Symptom-Complexes		Chief Symptoms for Differentiation	Approach to Treatment
Taiyang (cont.)	Symptom-complex of the fu organs	Stagnated blood accumulated in the channel	Fullness in the lower abdomen Incontinence of urine Mania Purplish tongue Deep and choppy pulse	Activate blood circulation to eliminate blood stasis
	Symptom-complex of the channel	Hyperactivity of dry-heat	High fever Extreme thirst Profuse sweating Dry, yellow tongue coating Overflowing pulse	Clear heat and induce production of fluid
Yangming		Heat accumulated in the intestines	Distending pain Fullness in the abdomen aggravated by pressure Constipation Dry yellow or dark yellow coating with prickles on the tongue Deep and full pulse	Eliminate dryness and remove accumulated heat
Shaoyang	Disorder of both the exterior and interior		Alternating spells of fever and chills Fullness in the chest and poor appetite Nausea bitter taste in the mouth Dry throat Blurred vision Thin, pale tongue coating Taut pulse	Remove pathogenic factors from Shaoyang channel

Channel	Symptom-Complexes	Chief Symptoms for Differentiation	Approach to Treatment
Taiyin	Discomfiture of spleen yang	Fullness and distending pain in the abdomen, eased by pressure Poor appetite Vomiting Diarrhea Pale tongue white coating Slow and weak pulse	Warm the spleen and stomach and dispel the cold from them
	Emerging cold symptom-complex	Aversion to cold Lying with body curled up Cold limbs Diarrhea with fluid stools containing undigested food Pale tongue with white coating Deep and feeble pulse	Restore yang from collapse
Shaoyin	Emerging heat symptom-complex	Restlessness Insomnia Dry mouth and throat Red tongue tip Deep, thready and rapid pulse	Nourish yin and clear up heat

TABLE 8.19. (*Continued*)

Channel	Symptom-Complexes	Chief Symptoms for Differentiation	Approach to Treatment
Jueyin	Symptom-complex of acute abdominal pain with cold limbs due to ascariasis	Intermittent severe abdominal pain around umbilicus, or pain in right upper abdomen Vomiting, or vomiting of round-worms Cold limbs; diarrhea; restlessness Red spots on the tongue Feeble and hidden pulse	Eliminate ascarides and reduce pain with drugs cool or warm in nature
	Deficiency of blood accompanied by cold limbs	Cold limbs Abdominal pain Vomiting Pale tongue with white tongue coating Feeble and faint pulse	Nourish blood, promote normal functioning of the channels, and dispel cold from the channels

Symptom-complexes of the first three are known as symptom-complexes of the *yang* channels; those of the last three are symptom-complexes of the *yin* channels. All of them reflect pathological changes in the *zang* and *fu* organs and the Twelve Principal Channels, respectively. However, the main purpose of differentiating symptom-complexes according to these six pairs is to analyze the changes due to exogenous pathogenic factors and their patterns of transmission.

Exogenous pathogenic factors can lead to symptom-complexes of the exterior, the interior, and both the exterior and the interior. The affliction of the six pairs of channels indicates where the disease is located. For example, disorders of the Hand and Foot Channels of Taiyang indicate exterior symptom-complexes; those of the Yangming channels refer to interior symptom-complexes; and those of the Shaoyang indicate a symptom-complex of both the exterior and interior.

Symptom-complexes of the three *yang* pairs of channels, even though caused by exogenous cold, often correspond to conditions of excess heat, marked by strong body resistance and hyperactivity of the pathogenic factors; disorders of the three pairs of *yin* channels often indicate deficiency symptom-complexes of cold, with a weakening or failure of the antipathogenic *qi*.

The analysis of signs and symptoms of the Six Channels thus allows the practitioner to further understand and confirm the diagnosis made on the basis of the Eight Guiding Principles. In addition, it suggests the possible path of development of the disease. Because the channels are all interconnected, it is possible that a disorder may be transmitted from one to the other. The practitioner can watch for signs of this transmission—a symptom-complex of one channel may be replaced by that of another, or symptom-complexes of two channels may occur simultaneously and thereby track the path of the disease.

Table 8.19 outlines the distinguishing features of the symptom-complexes of each of the six pairs of channels.

WEI, QI, YING, AND XUE

During the Qing Dynasty (1644–1911), a distinguished Chinese physician named Ye Tianshi introduced a theory of the *wei, qi, ying,*

TABLE 8.20. Differentiation of Symptom-Complexes in Accordance with the Theory of the Wei, Qi, Wing, Xue Systems

Stage of Disease	Symptom-Complex	Manifestations	Principle of Treatment
Disorders in the *wei* system	Invasion of the exterior by pathogenic heat (heat in the exterior)	Fever/ Slight intolerance to wind and cold/ Thirst/ Headache/ Coughing/ Sore throat/ Reddening of sides and tip of tongue with a thin, white coating/ Floating and rapid pulse	Dispel pathogenic heat from the exterior of the body with drugs pungent in flavor and cool in nature
Disorders in the *qi* system	Blockage of the lung by pathogenic heat	Fever/ Restlessness/ Thirst/ Coughing with asthmatic breathing/ Reddened tongue with yellow coating/ Rapid pulse	Clear pathogenic heat to ventilate and smooth trouble in lung
	Disturbance of the diaphragm by pathogenic heat	In mild cases: Fever/ Fidgeting/ Depression/ Fullness in chest/ Nausea. Severe cases: Continuous high fever/ Thirst/ Restlessness/ Burning sensation in diaphragm/ Dry lips/ Sore throat/ Constipation/ Concentrated urine/ Yellow tongue coating/ Floating slippery and rapid pulse	Clear pathogenic heat and ease the mind, or remove intense heat by purgation

	Hyperactivity of stomach fire	High fever/ Extreme thirst/ Profuse sweating/ Yellow and dry tongue coating/ Overflowing pulse	Clear pathogenic heat and improve secretion
	Accumulation of heat in the intestines	Fever/ Aversion to heat/ Delirium/ Fullness and pain in abdomen/ Aggravated by pressure/ Constipation; Yellow and dry tongue coating or brown coating with prickles on the tongue/ Deep and full pulse	Clear pathogenic heat by purgation
	Accumulation of damp-heat in the Triple Burner	Mild fever/ Perspiration with no alleviation of fever/ Fullness in chest/ Abdominal distension/ Loose stools/ Urine with red tinge/ Yellow, slimy tongue coating/ Rapid and soft pulse	Remove pathogenic heat and eliminate dampness with febrifugal and diuretic drugs/ Remove turbidity with aromatic drugs
Disorders in the *ying* system	Impaired fluid in the blood due to excessive heat	Fever or high fever at night/ Dry mouth/ Little thirst/ Fidgeting/ Insomnia/ Faintly visible rashes on skin/ Deep red tongue/ Thready and rapid pulse	Dispel pathogenic heat from the *ying* system with febrifugal drugs
	Invasion of the pericardium by heat	High fever/ Delirium/ Rigid tongue/ Cold limbs/ Deep red tongue/ Slippery and rapid pulse	Remove pathogenic heat to bring patient out of coma

TABLE 8.20. *(Continued)*

Stage of Disease	Symptom-Complex	Manifestations	Principle of Treatment
Disorders in the *xue*	Escape of blood from the vessels due to intense heat	Burning sensation/ Restlessness/ Delirium in severe cases/ Skin rash/ Expectoration of blood/ Epistaxis and bloody stools/ Dark purplish tongue/ Rapid pulse	Dispel pathogenic heat from blood and eliminate blood stasis
	Blazing of pathogenic heat in the *qi* and *xue* systems	Continuous high fever/ Restlessness/ Mania/ Delirium/ Hemoptysis/ Epitaxis/ Skin rash/ Expectoration of blood/ Deep red tongue with dry yellow coating/ Floating and rapid or deep rapid pulse	Clear and dispel pathogenic heat from the *qi* and *xue* systems
	Impairment of *yin* and stirring of endogenous wind	Slight fever/ Gaunt form/ Slight tremor or spasm of the limbs/ General lassitude/ Deep red tongue with scanty saliva/ Empty and rapid pulse	Nourish *yin* to subdue endogenous wind

and *xue* systems as a method of identifying symptom-complexes due to exogenous pathogenic heat. This method complements the method of differentiating symptom-complexes according to the Six Channels.

The essential distinctions in this method are:

—Symptom-complexes of the *wei* system involve attacks on the body's superficial defensive system by exogenous heat.
—Symptom-complexes of the *qi* system involve attacks on the seconary defense system by heat.
—Symptom-complexes of the *ying* system indicate an attack on the nutrient system by heat.
—Symptom-complexes of the *xue* system involve an attack on the blood system by heat.

These distinctions among symptom-complexes not only indicate four types of disease, but also the progressive stages of infectious diseases. Usually, the disease progresses from the *wei* to the *qi* to the *ying* and finally to the *xue* system.

The chief symptoms and treatments for each of these symptom-complexes are summarized in Table 8.20.

THE TRIPLE BURNER

The theory of the Triple Burner, developed by Wu Jutong during the Qing Dynasty (1644–1911), is a means of differentiating symptom-complexes of damp-heat in cases of infectious disease.

Epidemic infectious diseases are of two types: Warm-heat and damp-heat. While both types share symptoms of exogenous heat, dampness is the primary pathogenic factor in symptom-complexes of damp-heat.

Dampness is most likely to impair *yang qi*. It tends to linger between the *wei* and *qi* systems—that is, it has the characteristic symptoms of those symptom-complexes. It seldom invades the *ying* and *xue* systems without being transformed to dryness. Therefore, damp-heat is unlikely to impair the body's *yin*.

The diseases caused by pathogenic damp-heat are believed to result from the penetration of damp-heat throughout the Triple Burner. This presence of damp-heat in the Triple Burner blocks the normal

TABLE 8.21   Differentiation of Symptom-Complexes Due to Damp-Heat
in Accordance with the Theory of the Triple Burner

Symptom-Complex	Chief Symptoms for Differentiation	Treatment
Damp-heat in the upper burner	Aversion to cold/ Slight fever or absence of fever/ Afternoon fever/ Heavy head/ Lassitude/ Fullness in the chest/ Absence of perspiration/ Stickiness in the mouth/ Absence of thirst/ Fullness in the stomach region/ Lack of appetite/ Nausea/ Borborygmus/ Loose stools/ White slimy tongue coating/ Soft and slow pulse	Warm the exterior of the body and dispel dampness, or disperse damp-heat
Damp-heat in the middle burner	Mild fever that is relieved after sweating but reappears soon, or high fever in the afternoon/ General sluggishness/ Fullness in the chest and stomach region/ Nausea/ Lack of appetite/ Thirst with no desire for beverages/ Sallow complexion/ Delirium/ Concentrated urine/ Loose stools/ Pale and yellow tongue coating/ Soft and rapid pulse	Clear dampness and heat and promote the normal flow of *qi*
Damp-heat in the lower burner	Difficulty in urination/ Thirst with little desire for beverages/ Constipation or loose stools/ Distension in the lower abdomen/ Dizziness/ Pale or yellow slimy tongue coating/ Soft and rapid pulse	Eliminate heat and dampness with febrifugal and diuretic or cathartic drugs

flow of *qi* and injures *yang qi,* ultimately disrupting water metabolism. Wu's theory of the Triple Burner distinguishes three types of symptom-complexes based on the location of damp-heat in the upper, middle, and lower burners. Table 8.21 lists the characteristic symptoms of each of these symptom-complexes, along with their treatment.

THE CHANNEL SYSTEM

The theory of the channel system, described in detail in chapter 4, provides an auxiliary method for differentiating symptom-complexes in cases of internal disorders.

As the various channels follow their course of circulation on the exterior or in the interior of the body, they connect with and communicate to the *zang* and *fu* organs, respectively. They therefore reflect the condition of the internal organs along their course.

Differentiating symptom-complexes according to the theory of the channel system begins with the identification of symptoms—such as pain or impaired motion—that appear in specific parts of the body through which a channel passes. The relationship of this symptom to a particular organ is then analyzed along with other information to arrive at the proper symptom-complex.

While this method of differentiating symptom-complexes is subordinate to the other approaches to diagnosis, it provides direct guidance to treatment, especially by acupuncture and remedial massage.

For a review of the principal symptoms associated with each of the channels, see chapter 4.

THE ETIOLOGY OF DISEASE

No symptom-complex ever occurs without a reason. A symptom-complex is a reflection of pathological changes that are occurring in the body. These pathological changes, in turn, are responses of the body to a pathogenic factor. By understanding the potential pathogenic factors and their typical effects on the body, the traditional Chinese practitioner can trace the cause of a disease through the process of differentiating symptom-complexes.

The symptom-complexes that describe the effects of the various pathogenic factors are detailed in Table 8.22.

DIFFERENTIATING SYMPTOM-COMPLEXES AND DIAGNOSING DISEASE

The differentiation of symptom-complexes is the foundation of clinical practice in traditional Chinese medicine. It is a way of viewing disease—a way that focuses more on the process of change in the body and the relationship between these changes than on any specific disease agent and its behavior. it is a dynamic view of disease.

In its emphasis, diagnosis in traditional Chinese medicine thus

TABLE 8.22. Differentiation of Symptom-Complexes According to the Pathogenic Factors

Etiology	Symptom-Complex			Chief Symptoms for Differentiation
Wind	Exogenous wind	Attack by wind		Fever/ Aversion to wind/ Perspiration/ Scratchy throat/ Cough/ Nasal obstruction/ Thin white tongue coating/ Floating pulse
		Wind-cold		Aversion to cold/ Fever/ Headache/ Aching joints/ Thin and white tongue coating/ Floating and tight pulse
		Wind-heat		Fever/ Slight intolerance of wind and cold/ Headache/ Red eyes/ Yellow nasal discharge/ Sore throat/ Thirst/ Yellow urine/ Redness of the sides and tip of tongue/ Floating and rapid pulse
		Wind-dampness	In the exterior	Fever that is more severe in the afternoon/Perspiration that does not alleviate fever/ Aversion to wind/ General sluggishness/ Soreness in the limbs
			On the superficial portion of the body	Itchy skin characterized by oozing while scratching and by intermittent occurrence (such as tinea, eczema, nettle rash)
			Wind-like edema	General dropsy, especially marked by facial puffiness/ Swollen neck/ Difficulty in urination/ Aversion to wind/ Fever/ Cough/ Absence of thirst/ Floating pulse
	Endogenous wind	Wind stirred by liver yang		See differentiation of symptom-complexes according to the theory of zang-fu: symptom-complexes of the liver and gallbladder
		Stirring of wind in the liver by extreme heat		High fever/ Convulsions/ Rigidity/ Spasm/ Opisthotonos/ Deep red tongue/ Rapid and forceful pulse
		Endogenous growth of wind in the liver due to blood deficiency		Dizziness/ Twitching/ Tremor/ Pale tongue/ Slow and feeble pulse

Etiology	Symptom-Complex		Chief Symptoms for Differentiation
Cold	Cold in the exterior	Attack by cold	See symptom-complexes of wind-cold
		Direct attack by cold (on the spleen and stomach)	Pain in the stomach and abdomen/ Vomiting/ Borborygmus/ Diarrhea accompanied by chills and general aching/ White and smooth tongue coating/ Deep and slow pulse
	Cold in the interior (deficiency of *qi* with cold symptoms)		Intolerance to cold/ Affinity for warmth/ Cold limbs/ Watery vomiting/ Diarrhea with watery stools and containing undigested food/ Profuse and clear urine/ Lassitude/ Lying with the body curled up/ Cold and pain in the diseased body part/ Pale tongue with white coating/ Deep and fine pulse
Summer Heat	Attack by summer heat		Feverish sensations/ Profuse sweating/ Restlessness/ Thirst/ Preference for cold beverages/ General lassitude
	Heatstroke		In mild cases: Dizziness/ Nausea/ Oppressive feeling in the chest/ Vomiting. In severe cases: Unconsciousness/ Shortness of breath/ Profuse sweating/ Cold limbs
	Summer heat and dampness		Alternating spells of fever and chills/ Oppressive feeling in the chest/ Nausea/ Poor appetite/ Lassitude/ Loose stools/ Concentrated urine
Dampness	Dampness in the exterior	Wind dampness	See symptom-complexes of exogenous wind
		cold dampness	Impaired motion in severe cases of soreness and pain of the joints/ General aching/ Absence of perspiration/ Edematous limbs/ Oliguria/ Loose stools/ White slimy tongue coating/ Slow pulse
		warm dampness	Headache/ Aversion to cold/ Heavy sensation and aching in the whole body/ Suffocating feeling in the chest/ Loss of appetite/ Afternoon fever/ Absence of thirst/ Pale or sallow complexion/ White tongue coating/ Taut, thready or soft pulse

TABLE 8.22. *(Continued)*

Etiology	Symptom-Complex			Chief Symptoms for Differentiation
Dampness (cont.)	Dampness in the interior (accumulation of dampness in the spleen due to deficiency)			Poor appetite/ Stickiness in the mouth/ Absence of thirst/ Oppressive feeling in the chest/ Nausea/ Distension in the epigastrium and abdomen/ General sluggishness/ Lassitude/ Loose stools/ Diarrhea/ Edema/ Sallow complexion/ Turbid urine/ Leukorrhea/ Pale tongue with thick white slimy coating/ Overflowing pulse
Dryness	Dryness in the exterior	Warm dryness		Headache/ Fever/ Sweating/ Thirst/ Restlessness/ Dryness and pain in the nose/ Dry cough with scanty sputum or with bloody sputum/ Redness on the side and tip of the tongue/ Thin white and dry coating/ Floating and rapid pulse
		Cold dryness		Aversion to cold/ Fever/ Headache/ Absence of perspiration/ Dry cough with scanty sputum/ Dryness of the mouth and nose
	Dryness in the interior (consumption of fluid)			Dryness of the mouth and throat/ Dry, chapped skin/ Wizened hair/ Gaunt muscles/ Concentrated urine/ Dry stools/ Reddened tongue with little saliva/ Choppy pulse
Fire	Exogenous affection of epidemic heat			Early stage: Fever and slight intolerance of wind and cold/ Headache, sore throat/ Thirst. Second stage: Fever without chills/ Extreme thirst/ Restlessness/ Insomnia/ Delirium or stirring of wind and hemorrhaging when pathogenic heat invades *ying* and *xue* systems
	Internal growth of excess fire	Heart fire		Fidgeting/ Insomnia/ Flushed face/ Thirst/ Ulcers in the mouth and tongue/ Mania/ Delirium accompanied by difficulty in urination/ Urination with reddish tinge/ Pain in the urethra/ Blood in urine/ Reddened tongue/ Rapid pulse

Etiology	Symptom-Complex		Chief Symptoms for Differentiation
Fire (cont.)	Internal growth of excess fire (cont.)	Liver and gallbladder fire	Headache/ Dizziness/ Spells of ringing in the ears/ Flushed face/ Reddened eyes/ Bitter taste in the mouth/ Dry throat/ Burning pain in the costal region/ Restlessness/ Irritability/ Insomnia/ Dream-disturbed sleep/ Hematemesis/ Epistaxis/ Reddened tongue with rough, yellow coating/ Taut and rapid pulse
		Lung fire	Sonorous breathing/ Flared nostrils/ Expectoration of thick, yellow sputum/ Sore throat/ Thirst/ Preference for beverages/ Dry stools/ Concentrated urine/ Aching chest/ Expectoration of foul purulent sputum specked with blood/ Epistaxis/ Hemoptysis/ Reddened and dry tongue/ Rapid and slippery pulse
		Stomach fire	Burning pain in the epigastrium/ Acid regurgitation/ Stomach distress/ Thirst/ Preference for cold beverages/ Large intake of food without resolution of hunger/ Vomiting soon after eating/ Foul breath/ Painful gumulcers/ Hemorrhaging of the gums/ Constipation/ Reddened tongue with yellow coating/ Slippery and rapid pulse
	Internal growth of fire due to consumption	Stirring of fire due to *yin* deficiency	Feverish sensation in the palms of soles and the heart area/ Hectic fever/ Insomnia/ Night sweats/ Dryness of the throat and eyes/ Nocturnal emission
Seven emotional factors	Excessive joy (injuring the heart)		Trance/ Speaking incoherently/ Acting oddly
	Excessive anger (injuring the liver)		Pallor or flushed face/ Red eyes/ Fainting or syncope
	Excessive sadness (injuring the lung and spleen)		Emotional depression/ Poor appetite/ Cough/ Shortness of breath/ Abdominal distension/ Loose stools

TABLE 8.22. *(Continued)*

Etiology	Symptom-Complex	Chief Symptoms for Differentiation
Seven emotional factors (cont.)	Excessive pensiveness (injuring the spleen)	Poor appetite/ Lassitude/ Insomnia/ Amnesia/ Continuous violent palpitations/ Somnolence/ Gaunt form
	Excessive grief (injuring the lung)	Pallor/ Listlessness/ Grief and weeping
	Excessive fear (injuring the kidney)	Timidity/ Desire for solitude/ Listlessness/ Soreness in the lumbar region
	Excessive fright (injuring the heart)	Tendency to be easily startled/ Sudden palpitations/ Mental restlessness
Food intake	Dyspepsia due to irregular diet or overeating	Pain in the epigastrium and abdomen/ Poor appetite/ Fullness in the chest/ Vomiting/ Diarrhea/ Thick tongue coating/ Slippery and forceful pulse
	Food poisoning	Vomiting and diarrhea/ Oppressive feeling in the chest/ Colic/ Headache/ Spasms/ Irritability/ Delirium/ Salivation/ Difficulty in breathing/ Purplish face and lips/ Fever in severe cases
Work and rest	Excessive strain and stress	Listlessness/ Lassitude/ Feeble breathing/ Apathy/ Poor appetite/ Palpitations/ Fidgeting/ Mild fever/ Spontaneous sweating
	Lack of physical exertion	Obesity/ Shortness of breath after exertion/ Palpitations/ Dyspnea, weakness of the limbs
Phlegm	Wind-phlegm (stirring of wind due to excessive phlegm)	Dizziness/ Nausea/ Wheezing due to excessive phlegm/ Unconsciousness/ Facial paralysis/ Numbness of the limbs/ Hemiplegia
	Heat-phlegm	Expectoration of thick, yellow sputum/ Fever with irritability and restlessness/ Dry mouth and lips/ Dry stools/ Mania/ Yellow tongue/ Overflowing and slippery pulse
	Cold-phlegm	Thin and foamy sputum/ Aversion to cold/ Cold and pain in the joints/ Dark face and cold feet/ Impaired motion/ White and moist tongue coating/ Deep and slow pulse
	Damp-phlegm	Massive, thin and foamy sputum/ Easy expectoration/ Fullness in the

Etiology	Symptom-Complex			Chief Symptoms for Differentiation
Phlegm (cont.)	Damp-phlegm (cont.)			chest/ Poor appetite/ Nausea/ General sluggishness/ Lassitude/ Thick, slimy tongue coating/ Soft, slippery pulse
	Dry-phlegm			Sticky, scanty sputum that is difficult to expectorate/ Expectoration of sputum specked with blood/ Dry and painful mouth, nose and throat/ Dry stools/ Reddened tongue with little saliva/ Thready and choppy pulse
Fluid	Retention of fluid in the stomach and intestines			Vibrating sound in the stomach region/ Fullness in the chest/ Expectoration of thin sputum and saliva/ Absence of thirst or thirst with no desire for beverages/ Dizziness/ Palpitations/ White and smooth tongue coating/ Taut and slippery pulse
	Retention of morbid fluid (fluid in the chest and costal region)			Pain in the rib cage during coughing/ Distention in the costal region/ Dyspnea/ Deep and taut pulse
	Overflowing morbid fluid (fluid in the skin)			Heavy sensation and pain in the limbs/ Swollen limbs/ Difficulty in urination/ Fever/ Aversion to cold/ Absence of sweating/ Cough with asthmatic breathing/ Expectoration of massive, white foamy sputum/ White tongue coating/ Taut and tight pulse
	Raised morbid fluid (fluid above the diaphragm)			Cough with asthmatic breathing/ Fullness in the chest/ Wheezing/ Difficulty in lying supine/ Facial puffiness/ Foamy sputum/ Thick, white tongue coating/ Taut and tight pulse
Parasites	Round worms	Sallow complexion and wasting, poor appetite or even good appetite, preference for eating odd things, aching abdomen, potbelly		White spots on the face/ Blue spots on the sclera/ Red spots on the tongue/ Discharge of ascarids with stools or vomiting of ascarids
	Pin worms			Itchy anus/ Pinworms in the stools or in the anus
	Hook worms			Sallow complexion/ Puffiness/ Itchy eruptions on the skin/ Dark stools
	Tape worms			Stomach distress/ Continual feeling of hunger/ Separate worm segments in the stools

differs from Western medical diagnosis, which focuses on the disease agent more than on the efforts of the body to cope with the disease over time. The Western view, by comparison with the Chinese, is more static.

Contemporary practitioners of traditional Chinese medicine recognize the need for both views. They do not ignore contemporary Western knowledge of disease; they are, in fact, systematically integrating much of this knowledge into both their diagnosis and their therapy.

This integration follows a few basic principals. For example, when a disease has been diagnosed according to Western medicine, the practitioner will further classify the disease according to symptom-complexes, recognizing that one disease will produce different symptom-complexes at different stages. For example, a case of infectious hepatitis may manifest as: (1) the accumulation and "brewing" of damp-heat in the body; (2) a disturbance of the vital functions of the spleen due to external dampness; (3) stagnation of liver *qi;* (4) accumulation of cold-dampness in the body; (5) deficiency of both liver and spleen *qi;* or (6) insufficient liver *yin.* (These are not the only possibilities but are the primary symptom-complexes that occur with infectious hepatitis.) The disease is then treated according to the symptom-complex.

Sometimes, the Chinese practitioner will "abstain from symptom-complexes and treat the disease only." When a condition does not respond to the normal treatment for symptom-complexes, the practitioner will use a prescription developed specifically for the disease as it is diagnosed by Western medicine. (A number of herbal medicines have been developed to treat diseases by Western medical scientists in China.) The intent here is not to discard the Chinese theory; rather, whenever a cure is achieved in this way, the traditional Chinese practitioners attempt to establish new theories detailing the rules for combining the differentiation of symptom-complexes and the identification of disease.

If Western medicine is unable to diagnose the disease, the rule is to "abstain from the disease and treat only on the basis of symptom-complexes." Often a disease will be present, but a definite diagnosis cannot be made by present Western medical procedures and technology. In these cases, symptom-complexes can still provide an accurate guide to treatment even without a definitive diagnosis of the disease.

A fundamental principle of traditional Chinese medicine is "treating different diseases by the same method and applying different methods of treatment to the same disease." This principal, which has guided diagnosis and treatment through the centuries of Chinese medicine, is also appropriate when integrating traditional Chinese and Western medicines. Different diseases are treated alike when they manifest the same symptom-complexes; a single disease is treated differently when different symptom-complexes occur.[2]

Neither Western nor traditional Chinese medicine is complete in its approach to diagnosis. It is not enough for Western medicine to know only what a disease is; it must also strive to construct a complete picture of the disturbances in physiological functions as the disease develops. At the same time, Chinese medicine must try to integrate an understanding of the origin and behavior of the disease with its knowledge of symptom-complexes.

2. NOTE: Pathological changes can be considered the basis for this principle. For example, preliminary research suggests that the symptom-complexes identified as *qi* stagnation and blood stagnation are closely related to disturbances of the microcirculation. In light of this, these drugs are administered in such vascular disorders as coronary arteriosclerosis, obstructive cerebral angiopathy, retinal vein obstruction, thromboangiitis, erythema nodosum, and erythema induratum. These diseases all include the same underlying pathological problem—disruption of the microcirculation—and may thus be treated by the same methods.

GLOSSARY

Antipathogenic *qi:* the ability of the body to resist the invasion of pathogenic factors and to repair itself when those factors cause it harm.

Body fluid: a basic component of the body including, but not limited to, saliva, stomach fluids, synovial fluid, and tissue fluids as well as excretions. Its function is to keep the tissues and organs moist, to assure proper elimination of wastes, to maintain a normal body temperature, and to regulate the balance of *yin* and *yang* in the body.

Bo tie: the use of medicinal plasters.

Channel system: the energy network of the body. It links the exterior and interior parts of the body as well as the upper and lower parts. It joins the *zang-fu* organs and serves as the passageway for *qi* and blood.

Cun: a unit of measurement equal to about ⅓ decimeter. It is also one of the three positions on the wrist used for pulse-taking.

Defensive *yang:* see *wei qi.*

Eight Guiding Principles: also known as the Eight Parameters. These are the primary method for differentiating symptom-complexes. The eight principles are: *yin* and *yang,* interior and exterior, cold and heat, and deficiency and excess.

Endogenous pathogenic factors: pathogenic factors that arise from a serious internal imbalance.

Essence: also known as vital essence. it is the fundamental material of living organisms. Congenital or reproductive essence is received from one's parents. Acquired essence develops from food, air, and water following birth.

Exogenous pathogenic factors: pathogenic factors that come from the external environment. The principal exogenous factors are wind, cold, heat, dampness, dryness, and fire.

Five elements: the theory of the five elements is a theory of the process of change within a system. The process of change is described by analogy to the interactions among five basic elements: wood, fire, earth, metal, and water.

Five tissues: the skin, flesh, vessels, tendons, and bones. Each of these is related to one pair of *zang-fu* organs.

Gua sha: a procedure for treating sunstroke victims in which the patient's neck is scraped.

Lower burner: see **Triple Burner.**

Middle burner: see **Triple Burner.**

Nourishing *qi:* a rarefied substance transformed from food by the stomach and spleen to supply the body with nutrients.

Pathogenic factors: any harmful influences that disturb the relative internal balance of the human body or the balance between the body and the external environment. The literal translation of the Chinese *xie qi* is "evil *qi.*"

Original *qi:* derives from congenital and acquired essence and exists throughout the body, disseminated by the Triple Burner.

Pectoral *qi:* derives from air and food. It propels respiration and the beating of the heart.

Qi: the activity of life. It is described as a rarefied substance that circulates through the body, activating its functions. *Qi* is also the actual functioning of the body or parts of the body. For example, liver *qi* is the action of the liver in the body.

Qi **door:** refers to the pores of the body. It is the main pathway for the dispersion of body heat. The *qi* door is also referred to as the "mysterious house."

Symptom-complex: a complete summarization of the functioning of the body at a particular stage of an illness.

Triple Burner: refers to three parts of the body cavity—the upper burner, which houses the heart and lung; the middle burner, which houses the spleen and stomach; and the lower burner, which houses the kidney, urinary bladder, and small and large intestines.

Upper burner: see **Triple Burner**

Vital energy: see *Qi.*

Vital essence: see **Essence.**

Wei qi: sometimes called "defensive *yang,*" it defends the surface of the body against external pathogenic factors by opening and closing the pores of the skin, moistening the skin, and helping to regulate body temperature.

Xue: the *xue* system is the body's blood system.

Yin-yang: the theory of *yin* and *yang* states that any object in nature is a unified whole composed of two parts' with opposing qualities. These opposing qualities are described as *yin* and *yang.* Everything in nature can be classified as *yin* or *yang.* However, these classifications are relative. Thus, the *yin* or *yang* nature of an object may change in relation to another object.

Ying: the *ying* system is the body's nutrient system.

Ying and *wei* system: the defensive energy system of the skin.

Zang-fu: the *zang-fu* describe the internal organs of the body and their relationship to other tissues, to the sense organs, and to the channel system. The five *zang* organs are the heart, liver, spleen, lungs, and kidneys. The five *fu* organs are the gallbladder, stomach, small intestine, large intestine, and urinary bladder. The Triple Burner is also considered a *fu* organ.

INDEX